Bodybuilding Basic Training

The Absolute Beginner's Guide for Building Muscle

By

Brad Borland, MA, CSCS

Medical disclaimer

Brad Borland is not a physician or registered dietician. The contents of this manual should not be taken as medical advice. It is not intended to diagnose, treat, cure, or prevent any health problem - nor is it intended to replace the advice of a physician. Always consult your physician or qualified health professional before starting an exercise program or on any matters regarding your health.

Bodybuilding Basic Training

The Absolute Beginner's Guide for Building Muscle

What's included:

Section 2: Body Part Training   16

Section 3: Goals and Training Programs   147

What is this manual all about and who is it for?

Simply put, this *Bodybuilding Basic Training Manual* is for two main groups of people:

The absolute beginner

and

The frustrated and confused who are fed-up with their lack of building muscle.

Does either of these describe you?

This *Bodybuilding Basic Training Manual* is designed to give you a plan (more like many plans) to put on lean muscle. Nothing more, nothing less.

If you are a beginner or just want to wipe the slate clean and start from scratch, you are in the right place. *Bodybuilding Basic Training* cuts through all the crap and gets down to the basics.

Do you suffer from too much info?

With the countless bits of information out there on the internet it is easy to get confused, frustrated and downright angry by all of the different types of systems, programs and cool-sounding techniques.

You start to feel symptoms of *analysis paralysis*.

Here is what happens: Your goal is to pack on some lean muscle and you are hungry to learn all you can about training. So, you scour the internet for all you can possibly ingest wanting to know more and more about the latest, most effective training programs and tips. You keep searching and reading every last bit of information – one thing leading to another and another and another.

Soon, you find yourself paralyzed with so much info that you don't know which direction to go. All this research and no action leads you to become frustrated and with thoughts of throwing in the towel.

Does this sound anything like what you have gone through?

Take a deep breath and let's start over.

To start, two actions must take place.

First, stop reading so much. Stop the research, stop searching on the internet and stop questioning every tiny piece of information you come across. Simply put, stop and breathe. Clear your head and think happy thoughts.

Second, decide that it is time to pick a plan (one that is of sound quality) and stick to it.

If you decide to stop reading here and go with another plan – so be it. The important thing is that you decided to commit to a plan for a significant length of time – no hard feeling.

Still here? Great! Let's move on.

Packing on real, lean muscle is what you are after and so was I as a beginner.

At first I was a great example or "ignorance is bliss." I trained how I wanted to train, not caring a bit about what others were doing or what I read. The gains came (although it was tough and I put in a ton of hard work) and I was happy.

Then I started questioning everything, reading all the magazines and asking everyone in the gym their advice. I started down the path of information overload.

Guess what happened next?

My gains came to a halt. I no longer enjoyed training due to this wealth of knowledge, which I thought was a great thing.

Now, don't get me wrong, I love to read research and check out what the latest trends and practices are in fitness, but what good is sitting on the internet soaking up knowledge without putting it into practice?

I wrote *Bodybuilding Basic Training* with my "old self" in mind. I asked myself if I were to talk to the old me, what would I give him so he would be less confused, less frustrated and on a continued path of making gains in the gym?

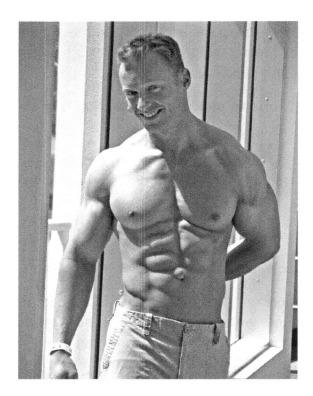

Bodybuilding Basic Training was my answer.

This manual will give you the basic tools of the trade without all the "tricks" and "special techniques" promising unrealistic and instant results in less and less time. This manual is about old-school, basic training designed to pack on real, lasting muscle the right way. Period!

How do I use this manual?

This manual is divided into three easy-to-follow sections:

Section 1: An Introduction to Training

This section is dedicated to explain some of the most commonly asked questions about the important parts of training. It breaks things down from reps to sets to rest and progress and much more. It answers your questions about the absolute basics of training, clearing up the confusion so you can get growing again.

Section 2: Body Part Training

This section breaks down each body part and some of the most common and effective exercises for muscle growth. Detailed explanation and countless tips about alternatives and simple, easy to use techniques for the best results.

Section 3: Your Goals and Training Programs

This section wraps everything together and gives you complete training programs specific to your goals. The programs listed are directly related to the exercises listed in Section 2. Simple, straightforward training programs – all that is required is your dedication and hard work.

Section 1: An Introduction to Training

Let's get down to basics. Let's talk a little about the guts of a successful training program to get you the best results possible. Nothing fancy here, just the absolute basic knowledge explained keeping it simple.

What is a rep?

The rep is the essence of any training program. Simply put, a rep is one complete movement of the bar, dumbbell or whatever you are using for an exercise. For your purposes, you will be using a cadence of two seconds of lowering the weight, two seconds of raising the weight and then a brief pause for contraction before repeating your next rep. Yes, there are countless rep cadences out there but a 2/2 ratio will best suit your needs and cut out confusion. **Simpler is better**.

What is a set?

A series of reps is referred to as a set. A set may consist of a single rep to as many as 100 reps. Many times you will see a formula such as 3 x 8 or 4 x 10 or any other combination. For example, 3 x 8 translates to three sets or eight reps each. After the series of sets is complete you will have completed a total of 24 reps.

What is a warm-up set? How do I warm-up?

A warm-up set is a relatively light set to "prime" the muscle and surrounding muscles with blood and to raise body temperature. If you were about to attempt a series of sets of the bench press, for example, and you were going to perform 4 sets of 6 to 12 reps (4 x 6-12) with 185 pounds your warm-up sets may look like this: set 1, 95 pounds x 15 reps, set 2, 135 pounds x 10 reps. After these warm-up sets, you are ready for the work sets.

What is a work set?

A work set is performed after your warm-up sets with a heavier weight. These work sets are the bread and butter of weight training. They are normally performed to the point of muscle failure to spur growth and change in the muscle or muscles being trained.

How should I breathe during a set?

Proper breathing is important during all exercises. You will want to inhale during all eccentric (lowering) of the weight and exhale during all concentric (lifting or exerting) of the weight. The act of the lungs filling and exerting will actually help you lift not only more weight but also stabilize your body for better form.

What is muscle failure?

Officially referred to as momentary muscular failure, it is the point at which after a series of reps you cannot perform another complete rep with proper form. At this point you will terminate the set. There is still a debate going on about if muscle failure is necessary or not, but most evidence points to achieving failure to give the brain the message to change the muscle to grow larger and stronger.

What is the best rep range to use?

Another heated debate brewing seems to be over the best rep range to use for maximum muscle gain. Some say low reps with the heaviest weight, others tout the advantages of higher reps with lighter weight.

The conclusion that I have somewhat come to over the years is to use a rep range from 5 to 20. Too broad you say? Well, to drill down to more specifics, the old adage of a rep range of 8 to 12 still holds true as well when talking about building muscle (remember, you want to build muscle and the shape of your physique – strength isn't your main priority). Most routines found here will be using the 8 to 12 rep range. However, the best approach is to utilize a variety of reps ranges from 5 to 20 over the course of any program. You may use 5 to 10 for several weeks then switch over to 12 to 16 for another few weeks.

Bodybuilding Basic Training covers all the bases when it comes to variety of rep ranges, scheduling the right times for change and challenging you for better, more efficient ways of packing on muscle. I have cut out the guesswork to give you the tools to focus on training and less time wasted experimenting.

How much weight should I use?

Determining the amount of weight to use can require a bit of trial and error – but don't worry about being exact. Most athletes and powerlifters use a percentage of what's called there one rep max (1RM). Since you are after building muscle and reshaping your body, use a trial and error method of finding the amount of weight to use as it relates to the rep range you are performing. When in doubt err on the side of caution and use a lighter weight and slowly increase the weight from there.

What is a pyramid of sets?

A pyramid of sets refers to a structure of sets that increases your working weight with each set while the rep count decreases. For example, a series of squats may look something like this: (weight x reps) 185 x 12, 205 x 10 and 225 x 8. Of course, the reps listed aren't set in stone. Your goal would be to perform as many reps as possible with proper form.

How do I progress?

The simplest way to progress is to have a goal of reps to achieve and then increase the weight slightly only when that goal is reached. Using our example above, if you have a goal of wanting to lift your heaviest weight for 10 reps before increasing the load then you could up your weight by 5 or 10 pounds. So, over time you now squat 185 x 15, 205 x 12 and 225 x 10 you would then increase the weight to look like this: 195 x 12, 215 x 10 and 235 x 8. Notice the reps scheme goes back down to the original structure of 12, 10 and 8.

How much rest between sets?

The amount of rest can vary greatly depending on your goals. For example, powerlifters and Olympic lifters require greater amounts of rest than that of bodybuilders and other athletes wishing to increase their muscle mass and reshape their physiques. For your purposes, the best rule of thumb is to rest one minute between sets for smaller body parts such as calves, shoulders, arms and other single joint exercises that require smaller amounts of muscle and two minutes for larger body parts such as back, chest and thighs. This can vary a bit but one and two minute rests keep things simple but effective.

What is the difference between compound and isolation exercises?

Simply put, a compound exercise is a movement that requires more than one joint to lift the weight. The bench press, for example, uses the shoulder, elbow and (to a lesser degree) the wrist joints. All work in unison to help lift the bar. An isolation exercise is one that only requires a single joint to move the weight. A barbell curl is a good example utilizing only the elbow joint. Compound exercises are normally your bigger lifts that move more weight and pack on more muscle.

What are supersets and other techniques listed?

There aren't tons of intensity techniques list in this manual for good reason – to keep things simple. But a few are thrown in every now and then.

Supersets: Two sets done back-to-back without rest. Once both sets are completed a short rest period may take place.

Trisets: A type of superset where three sets are done without rest in the same manner as above.

Giant sets: Another superset where more than three sets are performed back-to-back without rest.

Pre-exhaustion: When as isolation move for a certain body part is performed before a compound move. For example, a fly exercise is done before a bench press. The fly isolates the chest working mainly the pecs and then the bench press is performed after to push the chest further into muscular failure. Pre-exhaustion is often done for body parts that are stubborn to grow.

What about frequency, volume, intensity, duration and other factors related to my goals?

Bodybuilding Basic Training takes the guess work out of trying to structure the right training plan. Section 3 goes into detail about setting up the best program related to your goals. Frequency, volume, intensity and many other factors are worked out for you. Again, **simpler is better** and the plans laid out in this manual will get you there without confusion and frustration.

What about soreness?

A lot is still unknown about soreness but more and more research is being done every day. Currently, soreness isn't seen as a requirement for progress but many feel great amounts of soreness especially in the beginning of training. The flip side is also true: soreness is also not the greatest indicator as to signal you when to train again. Training a slightly sore muscle will not hurt your gains.

A word of caution: This does not refer to real injury to a muscle or joint. If you are seriously hurt, seek medical attention.

What about cardio?

Cardiovascular training is an important part of any exercise program. Not only to be used for fat loss, it is also an integral part of a healthy lifestyle. Having said that, this particular manual details structuring a physique-building program using resistance training. If cardiovascular training is to be performed it should be done after your resistance training or on a separate day.

I have more questions

If you have any questions, be sure to visit BradBorland.com for more on training, nutrition and motivation.

Happy lifting!

Section 2: Body Part Training

The Chest

The chest. It is, in many ways, what defines a man. A big barrel-like chest complete with muscularity, mass and balance exudes power, control and mastery over oneself. Most of us growing up as little boys looked up to our dads - they were bigger, stronger and taller than us. We were always impressed with their abilities to lift, pull, carry and push. Did we not look up to them with awe and inspiration? Did we not want to one day be like them?

The pectoral muscles are visually the hallmark of strength on the human body. They signify power and dominance in one's own personal space and beyond. Most men have at one point or another pursued a stronger and more massive chest in his lifetime whether they were the recreational lifter or competitive bodybuilder.

Although many of us spend countless hours on the bench press and pec deck machine, fewer and fewer actually build impressive muscularity in that area - instead we build monumental egos. We spend entire training sessions, sometimes lasting hours, and performing set after set of every movement known to man with little to nothing to show for it. Sure, we may become a little stronger and may gain a little muscle along the way, but wouldn't it be nice to work with a program that is both efficient and effective and produces respectable gains?

Hopefully this chapter will shed a little light on the infamously elusive greater pectoral development. This is not necessarily a strength program (although you will reap strength gains), but is a pectoral development program designed to increase muscle mass, development and balance from top to bottom, inside and out. To have a strong, well-rounded chest can put the finishing touches on any physique whether it is for the beach or the stage.

Anatomy and function

The musculature of the chest is comprised of two muscle groups. Let's take a look at each and there functions.

Pectoralis major: Located on the front of the ribcage, this fanlike muscle originates on the breastbone on the center of the chest and attaches to the humerus near the shoulder joint. The pectoralis major's main function is to bring the humerus across the chest.

Pectoralis minor: Located underneath the pectoralis major, this muscle originates on the middle ribs and attaches to the coracoid process of the scapula. The pectoralis minor's main function is to shrug the shoulder area forward.

Although the chest area is comprised of these two muscle groups, many exercises will influence different areas of the pectoralis major. Incline, flat and decline presses and fly movements will all affect this area in certain ways that can dictate development in one area over another. Additionally, the pectoralis minor, sometimes activated through stabilization purposes, can also be targeted for specific development.

Chest builders

Now that you know a little about anatomy and function, let's delve into what makes an outstanding chest. The movements presented are designed to get the most out of each trip to the gym. Remember to always use good form and not to use too much weight to compromise your safety.

Flat, incline and decline bench barbell, dumbbell and Smith machine presses: These groups of movements normally make up the majority of trainers' programs. The flat bench movements emphasize the middle and lower portions of the pectoralis major, the incline working mainly the upper and to a lesser extent the middle portion and the decline angle developing the lower "pec" area. These can all be performed with a barbell, dumbbell or Smith machine – each having their own advantages.

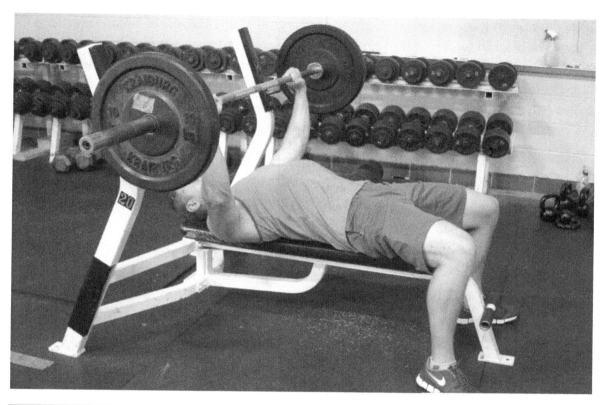

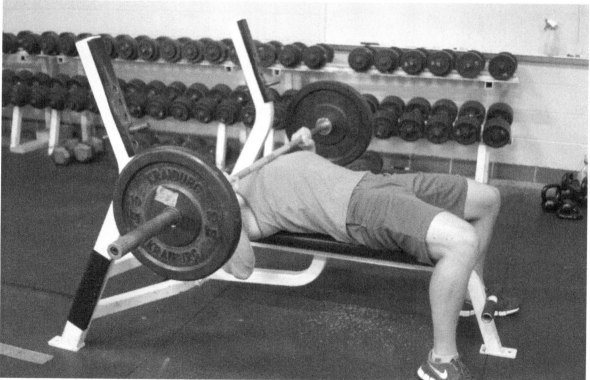

Barbells are normally utilized for maximum loads and overall mass and development. They are good to use at the beginning of a routine so that you can lift heavy amounts of weight early on in their program. Dumbbells have the advantage of being used in a unilateral manner in which you can not only even out imbalances from one side to the other, but also allows the pecs to work interdependently so that you can bring the dumbbells together at the top of the movement for a strong contraction. A Smith machine is best utilized near the middle or end of a routine when the joints have been fatigued and proper balance and form become an issue.

For barbell work, simply grasp the bar a few inches outside of your shoulder width (the best placement is a grip that positions the forearms perpendicular to the floor when the bar is lowered to the chest). Lower the bar to the upper chest for the incline version, mid to lower pec for the flat version and the lower pec line for the decline position. Without bouncing the bar, press the weight straight back up without locking the elbows.

For dumbbell work, execute the movement the same way but lower the dumbbells to the sides of your chest and then simultaneously press them back up and slightly toward the center without clanging the weights together. Be sure not to lock the elbows to keep constant tension on the muscles.

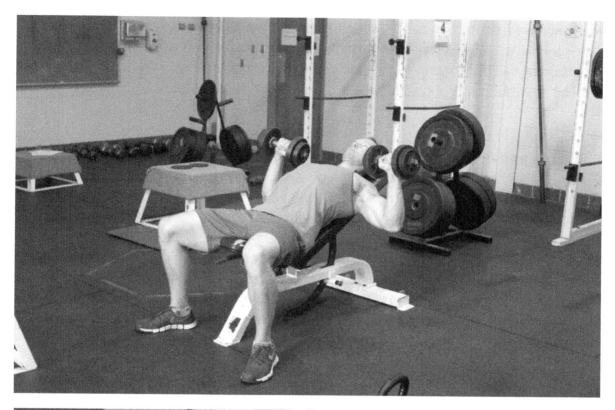

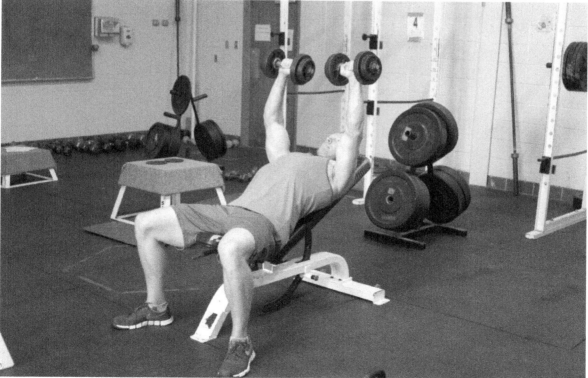

Tip: An often forgotten and seldom used pec-builder is the reverse grip bench press. Mainly utilized on the flat bench, the reverse grip press can also be performed on a

Smith machine (recommended). Grasp the bar with a reverse grip either at shoulder width or a little wider and have your training partner assist you with un-racking the weight. Lower the bar to your lower pec area and press back up in a controlled manner. Note: The reverse grip bench press is a great upper pec builder.

Flat, incline and decline dumbbell and cable flys: These movements will carve detail and fill out key areas of the pectoralis major – such as the inside (with cables) and outside (with dumbbells) of the muscle. Simply lie on a flat (for middle pecs), incline (for upper) or decline (for lower) with the dumbbells or cable "D" handles in your hands and your palms facing each other. For the cable version you will be using the universal cable machine and the pulleys in the lowest position. Expand out your hands as if you were about to give someone a giant hug. Your elbows should be slightly bent to relieve tension from your joints. Lower the dumbbells or "D" rings to about chest level (or a comfortable position) and then reverse the movement in the same hugging motion.

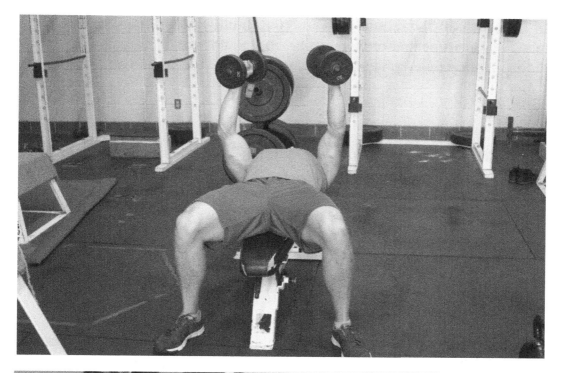

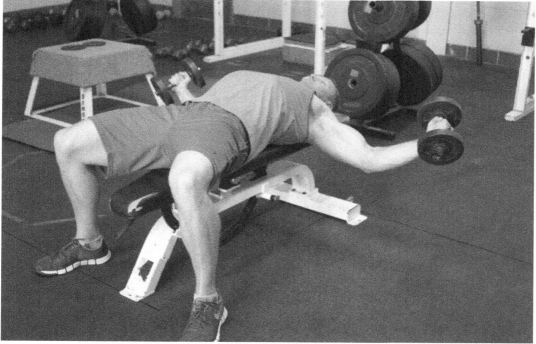

Tip: This is where the two pieces of equipment differ. While using dumbbells, do not touch the weight together at the top. Bring them together until they are about six to eight inches apart – this will keep tension on the pecs. For the cable flys, bring the handles together for an intense contraction and squeeze.

Hammer Strength and machine presses (flat, incline and decline): Most gyms have some version of the machine press. Just be sure to adhere to the guidelines as with presses described above – no lockout, slow on the way down and squeeze on the way up.

Machine pec deck: Another favorite of gym goers is the pec deck machine. These are usually found with the pads for the forearms or with the long straight-arm handles. The most important point to remember when performing these movements (which is similar to the fly motions discussed above) is to keep your shoulders back and expand the chest out at all times. This will ensure the pecs take more of the stress while protecting the shoulders. Be sure to squeeze for a second or two to increase muscle involvement and contraction.

Cable crossovers (high, mid and low): To get that deep inner chest development and an overall complete look to the chest, nothing beats cable crossovers. These can be performed in a variety of ways dependent upon what the goal is. For the traditional high pulley cable crossover grasp two "D" handles from cables that are set above your head and stand between the two cable towers. You will start with a slight bend at the elbow to relieve pressure from the joint. Step forward a foot or two and begin with your arms wide open. Bring your arms forward and down in a huge arc as if hugging someone with your hands coming together at about beltline level. Slowly return to the starting position by raising your arms in the same arc motion. This particular motion works mainly the lower and inner pec area.

Cable crossovers performed with the cables set at or around shoulder level will develop mainly the middle and inner pec area. Execute the motion the same way as described above; however, you will bring the handles directly in front of your chest instead. Squeeze and then stretch straight back.

With the pulleys set to the lowest position (closest to the floor), the low pulley cable crossover will help develop the upper and inner pec region. Again, start wide and this time low with the handles and arc them up until they are in line with your upper pecs or even your chin for an intense upper pec contraction.

Incline, floor and decline push-ups: Not just for boot camp anymore, this old favorite has made a comeback lately, especially amongst functional and group trainers. The push-up for most of us seeking a better pec landscape can normally be reserved for the end of a chest routine. Variations include: incline for lower pecs (hands on a raise bench and feet on the floor), decline for upper pecs (hands on the ground and feet on a raised bench) and floor push-ups for overall pec torture!

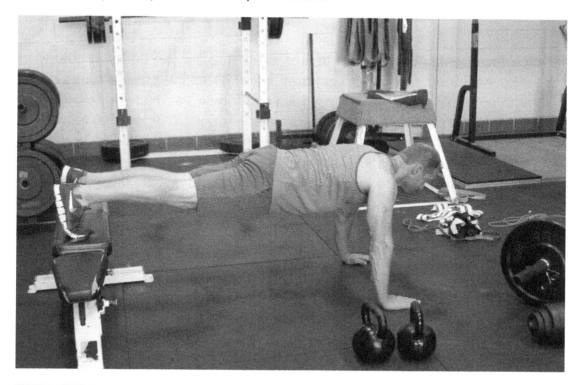

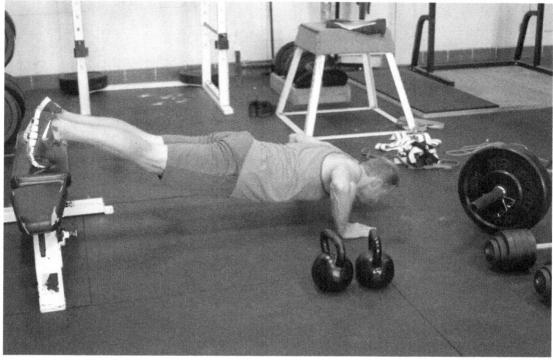

Tip: For even greater chest annihilation try performing a set or two of 3-way push-ups as your last exercise. Start with decline, then move to flat and finally incline with no rest between sets – that is one set!

Parallel dips for chest: Also used for triceps mass, the dip can easily be turned into a major chest builder. Step inside a dip apparatus and grasp the parallel bars about shoulder width apart. As you lower your body, lean forward and let your elbows flare out. You should feel a stretch in your pecs on the descent. While staying leaned forward, press back up focusing on the chest contracting. Weight can be added in the form of a dumbbell placed between your ankles by a training partner or by a weight belt with a chain to hold plates. Note: before adding weight, master the form first with just your bodyweight.

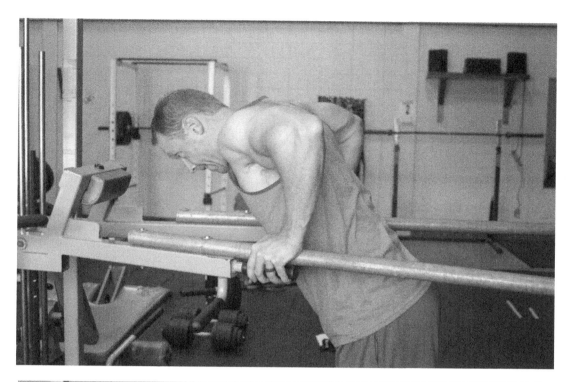

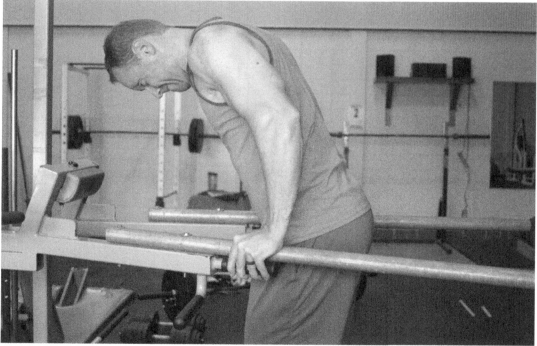

Dumbbell and barbell pullovers: Another great chest expander focusing on the pectoralis minor and overall depth is the pullover. Although many individuals utilize this movement for isolating the back, it is also extremely effective for "finishing off" the entire pec region.

For dumbbell pullovers lay perpendicularly across a flat bench grasping the inside face of a dumbbell of moderate weight. Start with the weight directly overhead and keep a slight bend in the elbows. Lower the weight back over your head in an arc toward the floor in a very controlled manner. As you lower the weight, take in a deep breath and stretch the chest. Stretch only where you are comfortable and then reverse the motion while blowing out. Remember: deep breaths will help contract the pecs.

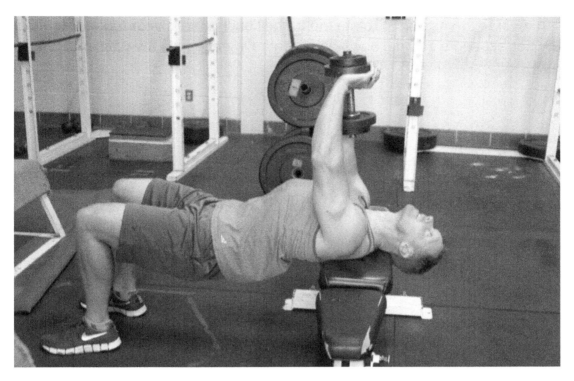

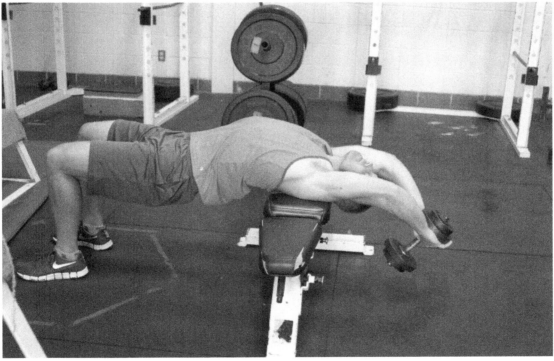

For the barbell version lie back length-wise on a flat bench and grasp a barbell slightly wider than shoulder width with a reverse grip. With the barbell on your chest (much like the bottom portion of a reverse-grip bench press) keep a 90 degree angle at the elbows. Rotate the weight up and over your head in an arc toward the floor. Feel a deep stretch and then reverse the motion to rotate the barbell back toward your torso. Remember to keep the correct angle at the elbows and breathe in deeply on the descent.

The Back

Not all of us will build a back of a bodybuilder but we can develop an impressive, V-tapered, thick and wide back that would not only turn heads but would also bring balance and strength to our entire upper body. You've heard of the term "strong back" and "put your back into it" – there is something to this.

The back comprises some of the largest muscles in the upper body from the lumbar to the trapezius and aids in almost every movement that we do from stabilizing our torso during the bench press to supporting the barbell during squats. The back is so important in our training yet few genuinely give it the attention it requires.

Many of us will do countless sets for chest, but neglect to put equal effort into our backs. One reason may be that it is difficult to see while standing in front of a mirror. Why train what you cannot see, right?

It does not surprise me to see so many in the gym with great big pecs, biceps and quads but little to show for back, hamstrings and triceps. Their shoulders are rounded forward because their pecs are pulling the deltoids forward giving them that concave look. The back has not been trained enough and/or correctly to pull the shoulders back and give a proper, proportionate look. The name of the game is balance. You must create that balanced mass and strength in order to have an impressive, muscular, strong physique. Having balance will enable other areas to improve and will help you avoid looking "front heavy" from the side.

Anatomy and function

With numerous muscles making up the back complex it can be a bit confusing as to which muscle does what, so let's take a quick look at what comprises the main muscles of the back.

Latissimus dorsi: Giving you that coveted V-taper, the "lats" make up most of the mass on the back. The triangular lat muscle extends from under the shoulders inserting from the humerus down to either side of the small of the back covering the lumbar region. Its main function is to pull the shoulders down and toward the back.

Teres major and minor: The teres major is a thick, flat muscle originating from the dorsal surface of the inferior angle of the scapula and inserts into the medial lip of the intertubercular groove of the humerus. It adducts and medially rotates the arms.

Rhomboid major and minor: The diamond shaped rhomboid major muscle which is located directly below the rhomboid minor inserts on the medial border of the scapula. It holds the scapula to the ribcage. Its job is to retract the scapula, pulling it toward the spinal column.

Erector spinae: These long muscles that run along the lumbar are divided into three columns: iliocostalis, longissimus, and spinalis muscles. They all work together to side bend and extend the spine.

Back builders

Now that you know a little about anatomy and function, let's delve into what makes an outstanding back. The movements presented are designed to get the most out of each trip to the gym. Remember to always use good form and not to use too much weight to compromise your safety.

Wide-grip and narrow-grip pull-ups: For the wide grip version use an extreme grip beyond shoulder width. Start with your elbows slightly bent and pull up to your chest focusing on cinching your shoulder blades together behind you. Arch your back and squeeze hard then return to the starting position with the slight bend in your elbows again. This will develop that sought after width and sweep in the upper lats.

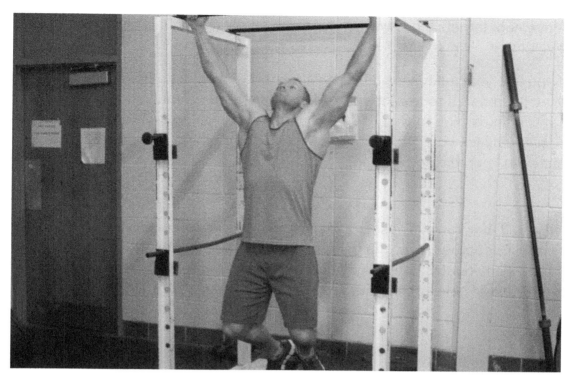

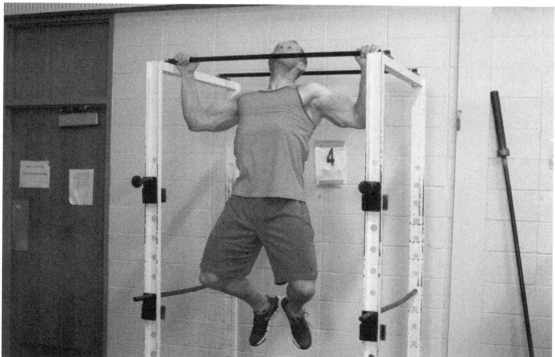

For the narrow version either grip the bar with a curl grip or with a parallel grip no wider than your shoulders, but at least six inches between your hands. Pull up in the same fashion as the wide grip pull up and lower yourself just prior to locking out your arms.

This movement targets the lower portion of the lat giving you thickness where it inserts near the lumbar.

Tip: If you find yourself having difficulty doing this movement a good trick I like to use is pick a total number of reps – let's say 40 – and try to reach that number no matter how many sets it takes. You may get 10 on your first set, 8 on your second, 7 on your third. Keep going until you total 40. When you are able to do three or four sets of 10 or 15 reps increase your total to 50 or so.

Barbell and T-bar rows: These are considered mass builders for the overall thickness of the back. For barbell rows grip the bar about shoulder-width. Bend over keeping your back in line with your hips and slightly above parallel to the floor, pull the weight into your stomach and squeeze the weight up. Lower the bar slowly and repeat.

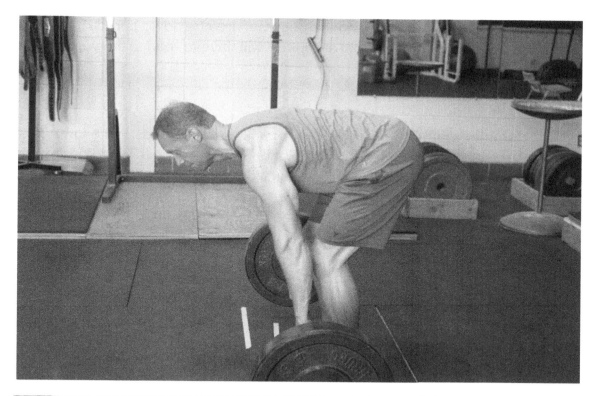

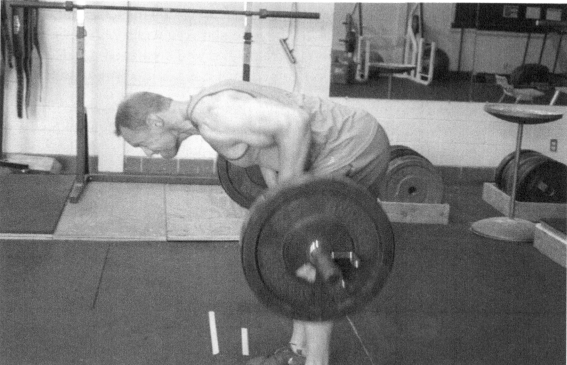

For T-bar rows follow the same guidelines but try not to throw the weight up and round your back. Keep a straight back and let the lats do the work not your lumbar.

Tip: If you find you are lacking mass in the upper lat area try doing barbell rows with a wider grip and pull into the lower chest area. You will have to reduce the weight to keep good form.

Pulley and Hammer machine rows: To really pack on some mass in the lower lat area near the lumbar try one of these on for size. For pulley rows sit with your knees slightly bent and upper body tilted forward. Simultaneously pull the handle back while straightening out your body to be perpendicular to the floor. Squeeze your shoulder blades together and pull the handle into your abdominals. Return to the starting position and repeat.

The beauty of hammer machine rows is that you can work one side at a time. Use the same principles as above and make sure to squeeze when pulling back.

Tip: If you ever feel uncomfortable doing barbell rows, affix a wide handle to a pulley row cable and do shoulder-width (or wider) pulley rows in place of barbell rows.

Parallel-grip and wide-grip pulldowns: Nothing hits the teres muscles quite like the parallel-grip pulldown. Grip a bar that is just beyond shoulder width with a slight bend in the elbows. Pull the handle down to the mid chest level and squeeze hard. Return to the top position feeling the weight pulling your lats up and out.

For wide-grip pulldowns grip the bar with an overhand grip and pull down to your upper chest level and return keeping your elbows bent and allowing your whole shoulder girdle to rise with the weight. These are a great substitute for pull-ups.

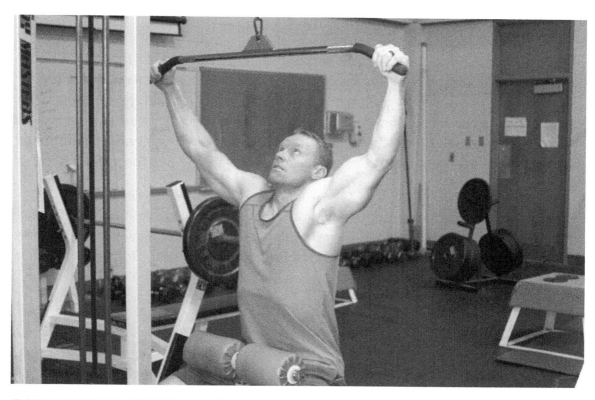

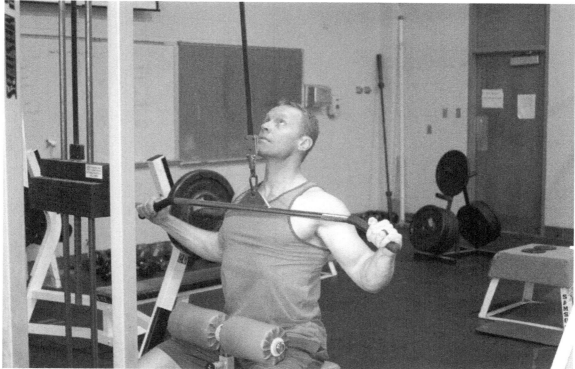

Tip: When doing any pulldown motion try raising your shoulder girdle in the starting position. As you pull down, lower your shoulder down and back and stick your chest out. This will ensure your back is fully engaged.

Dumbbell pullovers and lat pulls: As two of the very few isolation moves for back pullovers and pulls are great for finishing off the back. For dumbbell pullovers lay perpendicular on a bench with just your upper back in contact with the pad and your head hanging over the side. Grip the inside of a dumbbell directly over your chest with a slight bend at the elbow. Lower the weight back and behind your head in an arch until you are at least in line with your head and with your lats only, pull the weight back up to starting position.

For lat pulls stand in front of a lat pulldown or other overhead cable machine. Grip a bar shoulder width where the tension in on your lats about eye level. Pull the weight down to your thighs without bending your arms and squeeze the lats hard. Return to eye level with the bar and repeat.

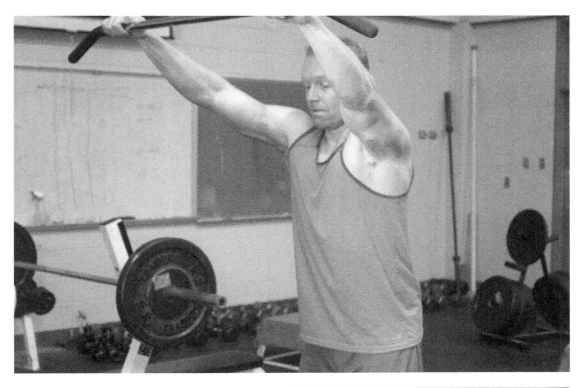

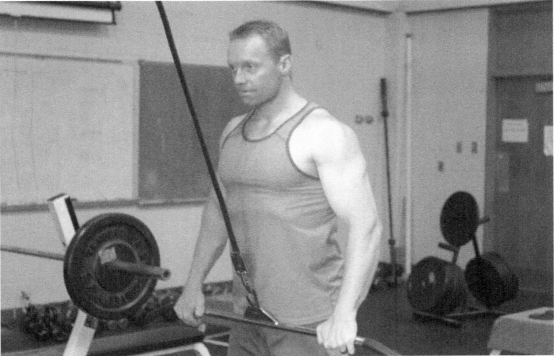

Tip: Either of these moves is great if utilized as a pre exhaust prior to the rest of your back work. A quick three sets of moderate reps will do the trick.

Deadlifts: The granddaddy of the back movements: deadlifts! This movement is for total head to toe thickness especially for the back. Load a bar on the ground and take a shoulder grip, bend at the knees keeping your back straight. Lift the weight off of the ground first with your legs and then straighten out you back until you are standing straight up. Return the bar to the ground in the same (but opposite) fashion.

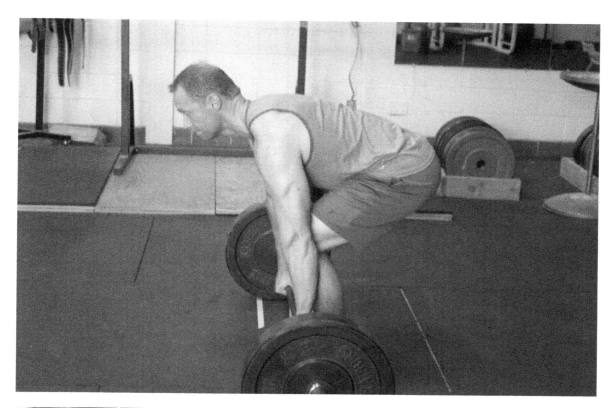

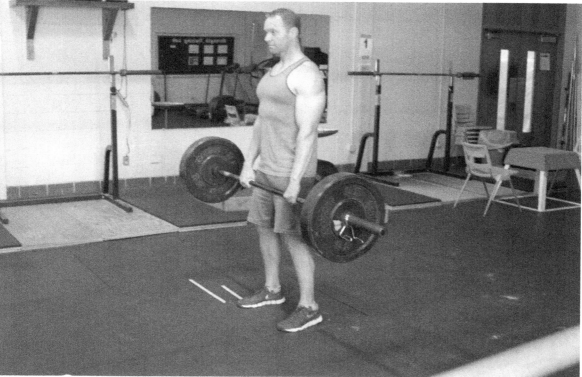

Tip: If you find yourself having difficulty doing off the floor deadlifts, try doing partial deadlifts. Load the bar on a bench that is just below knee level and follow the above lifting principles. This will take a little strain off of the back if you are taller or want to take some of the leg muscles out of the movement.

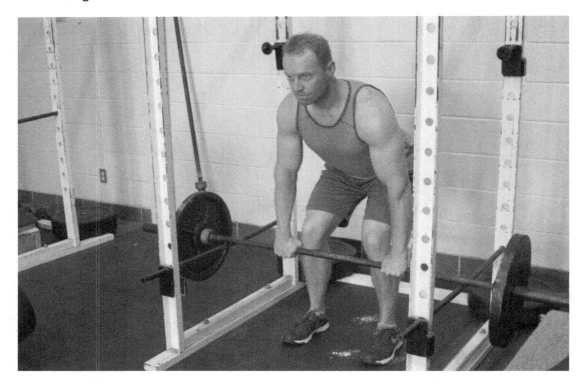

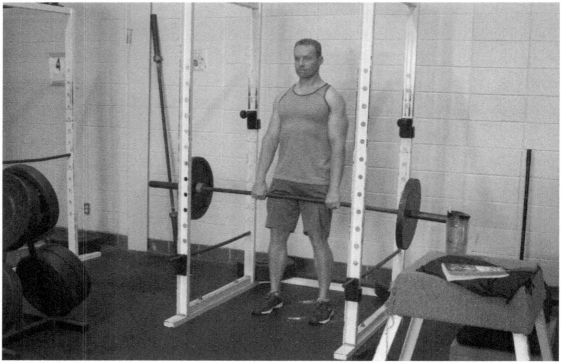

The Shoulders

We've all heard the saying: Sometimes it feels like you have the weight of the world on your shoulders. The shoulder region makes up a vital portion of our overall physique. Viewed from the front, side and back, the deltoids and trapezius muscles are essential not only to a well-balanced look, but also facilitate many other functions which synergistically work to produce results in other areas. Strong, well-built delts and traps go a long way in regard to making the entire body look strong and balanced.

Shoulders make you look broad and strong. Building proportionate delts and traps should be the goal of anyone looking to build the ultimate physique. One can often look at the shoulders as an integral piece of the infamous "X-frame" puzzle. If you were to draw diagonal lines from delt to calf, you would create the much sought after "X" physique. With developed delts and traps, a conditioned midsection, and well-built calves, your dream can become reality.

Take the time to dedicate some know-how, intensity and variety into effectively packing on some significant muscle to your "yolk" muscles. A carefully laid plan of action will help you on your journey to looking bigger and broader in less time.

Anatomy and function

With a muscle group as complex as the deltoid region it can get a bit confusing as to which deltoid head does what. With so many angles to choose from let's take a look at how they work.

Anterior deltoid: Originating from the collar bone and attaching to the humerus, the anterior (front) deltoid head raises the arm away to the front of the body. This deltoid head is heavily utilized in many pressing movements.

Lateral deltoid: Also originating from the collar bone and inserting into the humerus, the lateral (middle) deltoid head abducts the arm out to the side and away from the body. This head gives the upper body its wide look when developed properly.

Posterior deltoid: Originating on the scapula and inserting on the humerus, the posterior (rear) deltoid head moves the arm away and back from the body. The posterior head is strongly utilized in back movements such as pulls and rows.

Trapezius: This is a long, trapezoid-shaped muscle that runs along the upper section of the spinal cord, originating at the base of the skull and attaching in the middle of the lower back. The traps function includes scapular elevation (shrugging up), scapular adduction (bringing the shoulder blades together) and scapular depression (pulling the shoulder blades down).

Shoulder builders

Now that you know a little about anatomy and function, let's delve into what makes outstanding shoulders. The movements presented are designed to get the most out of each trip to the gym. Remember to always use good form and not to use too much weight to compromise your safety.

Military (barbell) and dumbbell shoulder press: Mainly working the anterior and lateral heads the military press can't be beat. Take a slightly wider than shoulder width grip and start with the bar just under chin level and press up without locking your elbows. Return to the start position. This should be one fluid motion without a long pause at the top of the movement.

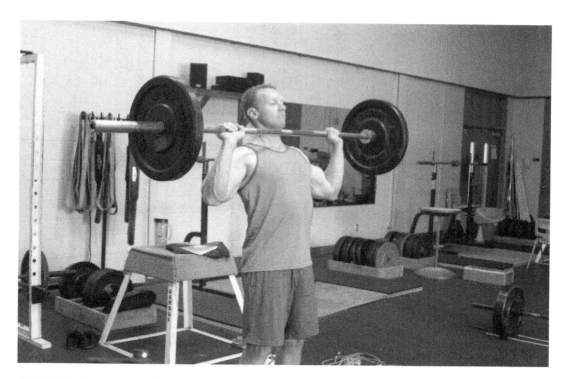

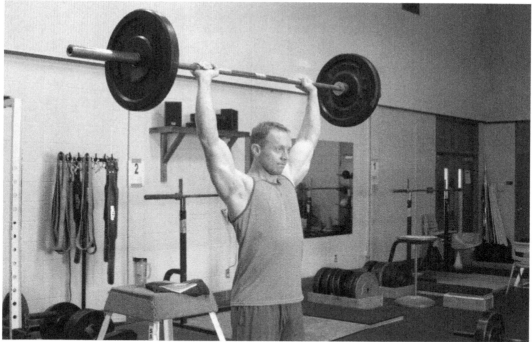

For dumbbell presses start with the dumbbells on either side of your head with your elbows flared to the sides. Make sure not to start the movement too high; start the dumbbells almost touching your shoulders. Press overhead simultaneously bringing the weights closer together at the top just short of locking your joints. DO NOT clang the weights at the top of the movement – this will cause a shock to the shoulder joints. Return to the start and repeat.

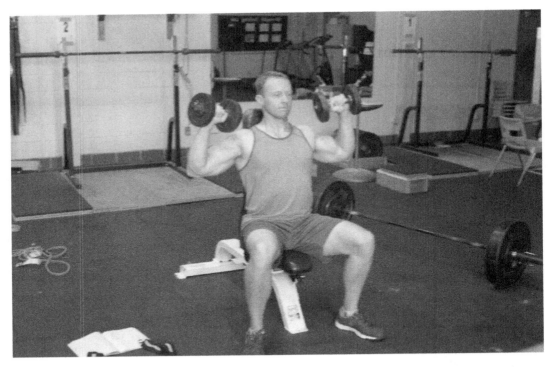

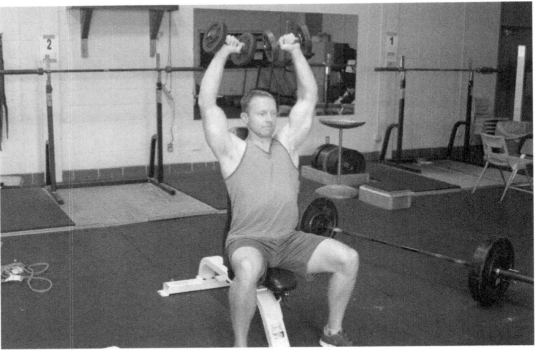

Tip: A great alternative and one in which requires less stability on your part is the Smith machine press. This machine allows for a greater amount of weight to be used due to the reduction of ancillary muscles required. Also, it allows for ease of racking and un-racking the weight.

Dumbbell and cable side lateral raises: To target the lateral head of the deltoid complex side laterals do the trick. When performing dumbbell side lateral raises (seated or standing) start with the dumbbells slightly in front of your thighs with a slight bend in your elbows. Here's the tricky part: you will not perform these as every other trainer has taught in the past (the ole "pour the pitcher of water" technique). You will bring the dumbbells out with the pinky in the up position the entire time. The thumb will be pointing down the entire time with no twisting. This isolates the lateral deltoid head to an extreme extent so use light enough weight to perform it properly. Return the weight the same way and repeat.

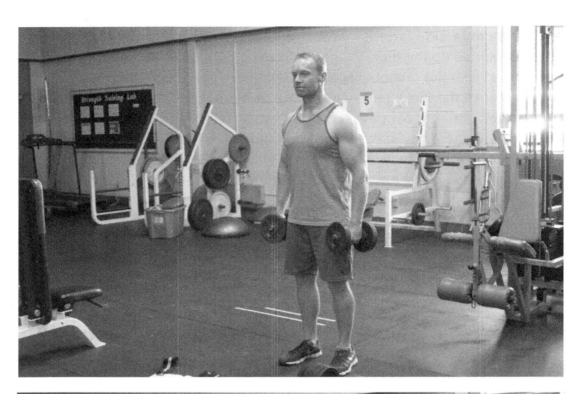

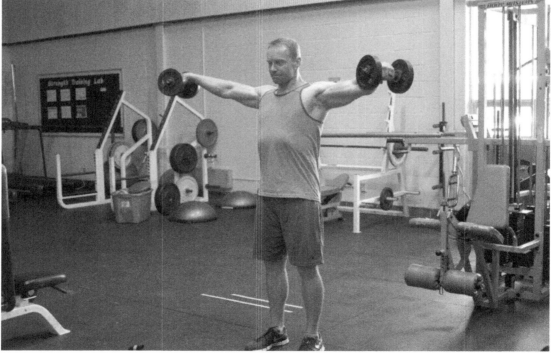

For cable side laterals stand next to the cable apparatus and grip a "D" handle with your distant hand (the one away from the cable machine). Start with the handle in front of you so your arm crosses your body with a slight bend at the elbow and raise the handle up and out until it is parallel to the floor. Pause and squeeze at the top and lower the weight slowly in the same manner. Performing for each side counts as one set.

Tip: A good change of pace would be to perform leaning one-arm laterals. Grip a dumbbell in one hand and grab a fixed upright in another. With your feet against the upright lean out to your side until your non-working arm is straight. Now the dumbbell is hanging at an angle from your body. Raise the dumbbell as you would the two arm version until your arm is parallel to the floor. You will notice that you actually are a little higher than shoulder level as with normal laterals. This will activate more deltoid fibers and isolate one side at a time enabling you to use slightly more weight.

Bent dumbbell lateral raises and reverse pec deck rear laterals: For the posterior heads bent dumbbell lateral raises can be performed standing or seated. Be sure when performing these bend over at the hips parallel to the floor as you would a Romanian deadlift and not the waist. Grip two dumbbells of moderate weight and begin the movement with a slight bend at the elbow and raise the weight up and out to the sides. Come parallel to the floor and return to the starting position without clanging the weight together. Try not to raise the weight up and back too much; this will transfer the load to the back muscles.

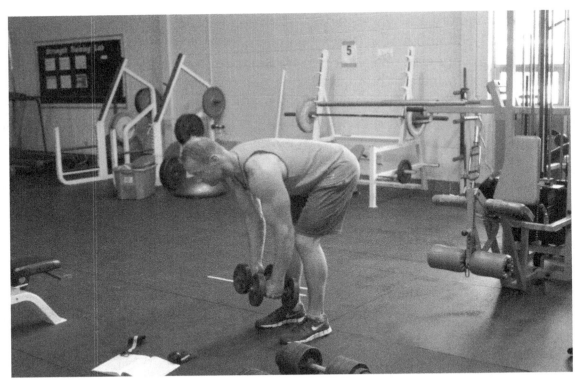

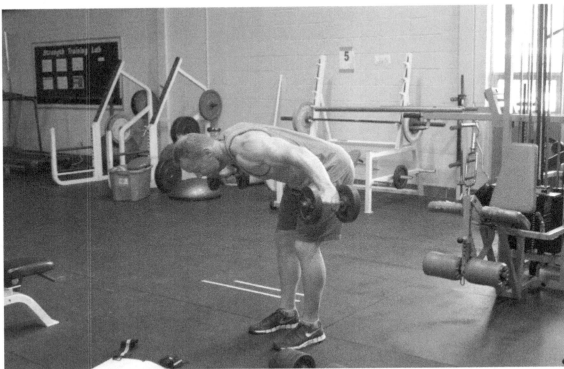

For reverse pec deck rear laterals set the seat of the machine so that your shoulder joint is in line with the handles. Grip the handles in either a palms facing each other or palms facing down position – whichever feels more comfortable. Pull the handles out and back until they are straight out to your sides and squeeze. Return the weight slowly to the starting position without letting the weight rest.

Tip: For a slight change and massive pump in the posterior delts try cable rear laterals. Stand in a cable crossover station and grip the cables (which should be set at shoulder level) with the opposite hands – grip the right cable with your left hand and the left cable with your right hand. This position should have your arms crossed in front of you. Take one step back so your arms and the cables can clear your body. Uncross your arms with a slight bend at the elbow and pull the weight back as in the bent over version. Squeeze your deltoids and slowly return the weight.

Barbell and cable wide grip upright rows: To ultimately get that overall roundness to the deltoids, especially the lateral heads, wide-grip upright rows are the perfect choice. Grasp a barbell with an overhand grip a few inches outside of shoulder width in front of your thighs. Pull the weight up along your upper body with elbows out until your upper arms are parallel to the floor. Squeeze the delts at the top and return to the start.

With cable upright rows simply attach a long bar to a low cable pulley and perform the same hand placement and movement as above. Utilizing the cables will give the muscle constant tension especially the squeeze at the top for a maximum contraction.

Tip: For those who have shoulder problems or find upright rows a bit uncomfortable and still want to reap the benefits of this movement, try some dumbbell upright rows. Hold the dumbbells in front of your thighs and pull the weight up as with barbell upright rows. The difference will be the freedom of arm movement which will alleviate some stress from the shoulder area.

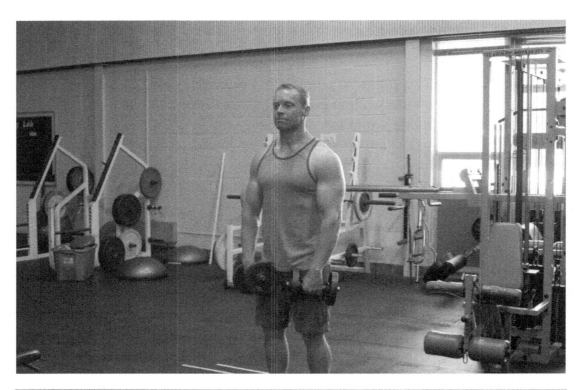

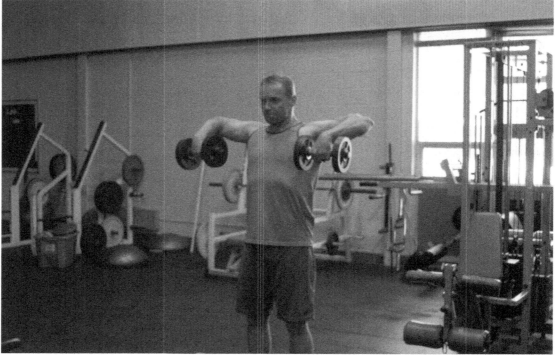

Barbell and dumbbell front raises: Used often as a great finishing movement for the anterior and lateral deltoid heads are front raises. Hold a barbell with an overhand grip about shoulder width in front of your thighs. With a slight bend at the elbows raise the bar in front of you at the shoulder joint only until it is approximately eye level. Return the bar slowly to the start position.

For dumbbell front raises hold two dumbbells by your side with thumbs forward. Raise the weights out in front of you at the shoulder joint only without twisting. Once you have reached eye level return to start.

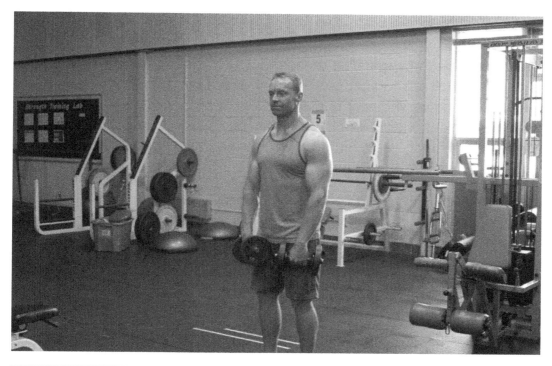

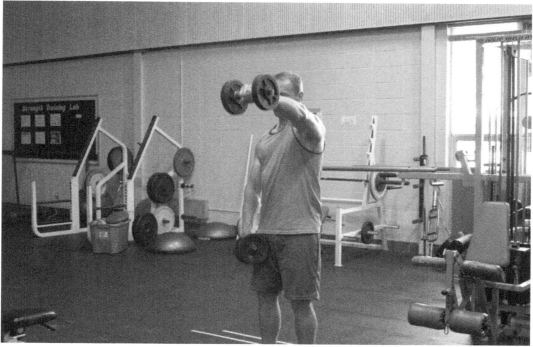

Tip: If your gym is busy and the weights are at times hard to get to or are being used another way to do front raises is with a weight plate. Plate raises are a convenient alternative to barbells or dumbbells. Grasp a weight that you can comfortably handle for your allotted reps as if you were holding a steering wheel. Make sure your grip is slightly on the underside of the plate so you can somewhat cradle it when you raise it. Raise and lower the plate as with dumbbell front raises.

Barbell and dumbbell shrugs: The granddaddy of trapezius movements is the barbell shrug. Grasp a barbell at shoulder width with an overhand grip against your thighs. Shrug up with your entire shoulder girdle reaching up to your ears and squeeze and slowly lower the weight back down. Important note: DO NOT rotate the shoulder during this movement. It is simply an up and down movement. Do not circle the shoulders forward or back; this can cause injury.

You may find dumbbell shrugs to be more comfortable and functional. Whereas a barbell is in front of you and can sometimes tip you forward, dumbbells are lifted from your sides and help with balance. Grasp a pair of dumbbells by your sides with your thumbs facing forward and shrug them straight up and squeeze. Return the weight back to start and repeat.

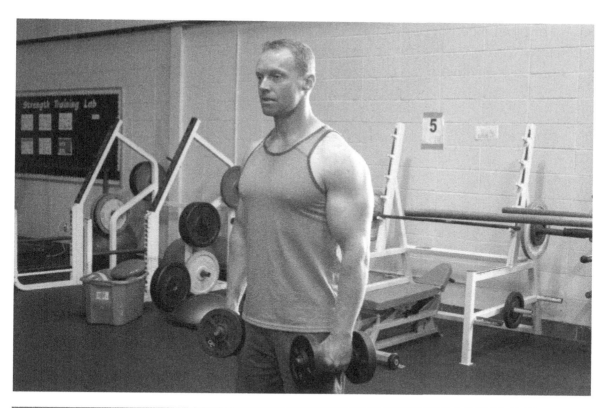

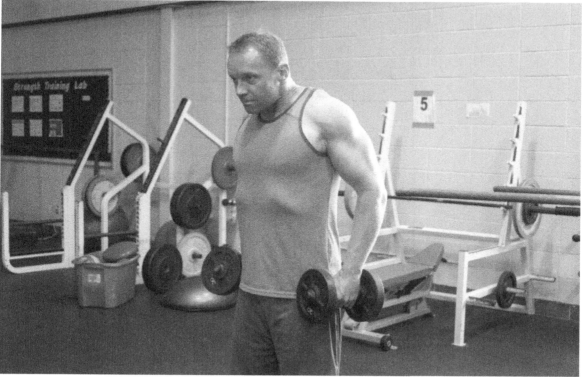

Tip: If your flexibility calls for it, a variation of the barbell shrug could prove to be beneficial. The behind-the-back Smith machine shrug is a great alternative to the traditional movements. Stand in front of a Smith machine and grasp the bar with an overhand grip behind your hamstrings and glutes. Step forward just a few inches so the bar can clear. Shrug the weight up as in a barbell shrug and squeeze. Your range of motion may be a bit limited, so be careful and maintain strict form.

The Triceps

Making up most of the upper arm mass, the triceps, once well developed, pay big dividends toward total arm mass. Unfortunately many of us fail to pay enough attention to this almost unseen muscle group instead spending most of our time on its next door neighbor, the biceps.

"Make a muscle!" I hear across the gym floor and inevitably I see a shirt sleeve roll up and someone is trying to flex their biceps peak while their triceps lies underneath ignored, underused, and underappreciated. Poor little triceps – and I mean little.

The triceps deserve better. All three heads demand the proper attention utilizing a carefully planned program and applied intensity.

As the antagonistic counterpart to the biceps, the triceps actually will directly aid in the development and strength of the biceps creating greater blood flow and nutrient uptake in the upper arm area. Your goal, therefore, should be to hit the triceps from all angles utilizing several movements and the right amount of volume. Well built, shirt-busting, horseshoe-shaped triceps will make any arm look balanced, proportionate and huge.

High and low reps, compound and isolation movements, volume adjustments, and angel selection should all be considered when structuring a sound program. With the right tools, know-how, and intensity anyone can move their triceps development to a higher level. So quit curling for just a few minutes and read on about the untold story of bigger arms!

Anatomy and function

The **triceps brachii** has three heads which connect the humerus and scapula to the ulna (in the forearm). The **lateral, medial, and long** heads make up the triceps.

The head that is most responsible for the horseshoe shape is the **lateral head** which is located on the outward facing side of the humerus. The **medial head** is located towards the midline of the body and the **long head** (the largest of the three) is located along the bottom side of the humerus.

Extending the elbow (straightening the arm) is the primary function of the triceps. The long head has a secondary function: it assists the latissimus dorsi in adduction of the arm (bringing the arm down toward the body).

Triceps builders

Now that you know a little about anatomy and function, let's delve into what makes outstanding triceps. The movements presented are designed to get the most out of each trip to the gym. Remember to always use good form and not to use too much weight to compromise your safety.

Cable pressdowns: No triceps program would be complete without the tried and true cable pressdown. Performed with a straight bar, V-bar, or rope attachment, pressdowns are invaluable to achieving that coveted "squeeze" contraction when performed correctly. Stand in front of an upright cable apparatus with a shoulder width stance. Grasp your chosen attachment with a firm grip and your elbows by your side. With your elbows stationary, press the bar or rope down toward your upper thighs and straighten your arms out to fully contract the triceps. Under control, return to the top position (make sure to get a full range of motion), making sure your elbows remain by your side. It is also important to keep proper posture during the movement by avoiding hunching over with your back. Maintain a straight and firm posture with the entire body.

A trick you may want to try is to imagine pressing the weight in an arch toward the wall behind you instead of straight down. This will ensure you will not use too much weight. Also, try different grip attachments. The straight bar tends to stress the larger inner long head while any movement with your thumbs pointing up as in rope extensions will work more of the outer head giving the horseshoe look.

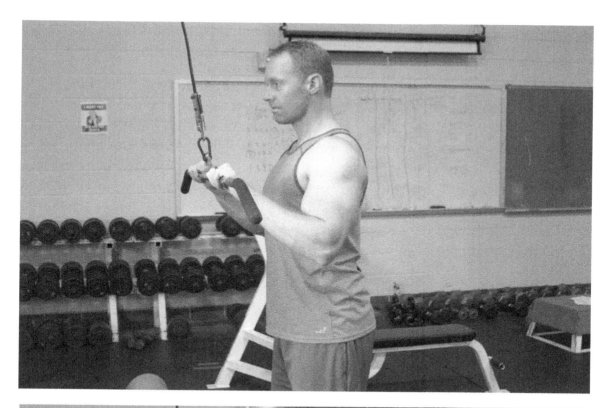

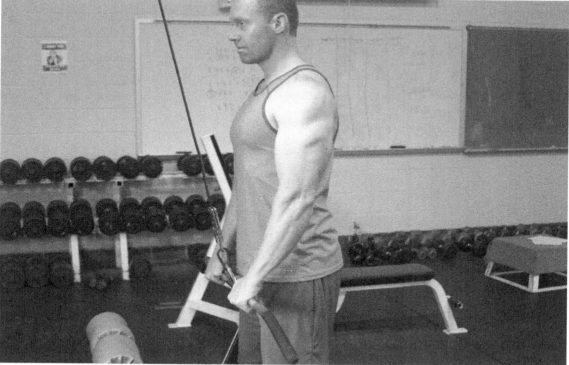

Tip: For maximum contraction without a lot of weight try reverse grip pressdowns with a cambered (EZ) bar. You will have to use slightly less weight, but the contraction is a killer! Grasp the bar as if you were going to do EZ bar curls (thumbs higher than your pinkies) and press down as if performing a regular cable pressdown.

Lying, seated, and standing French presses: The granddaddy of triceps moves is the lying French press (or more famously known as nosebreakers or skullcrushers). Simply lie on a flat bench with either a straight bar or EZ bar and extend the weight directly over your upper body with your arms locked. Angle your arms at the shoulder joint back slightly toward your head while maintaining the locked elbows. This will place constant tension on your triceps. To start the movement, bend only at the elbows and lower the bar toward the top of your head while maintaining that angle in your upper arms at all times. Stop the bar an inch or so above your head and then reverse the motion bringing the bar to the angled position once again straightening your arms.

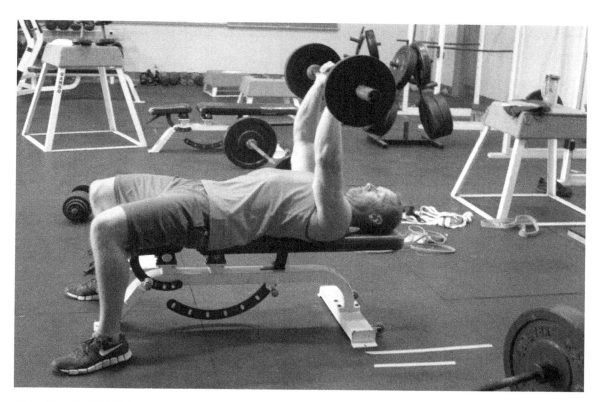

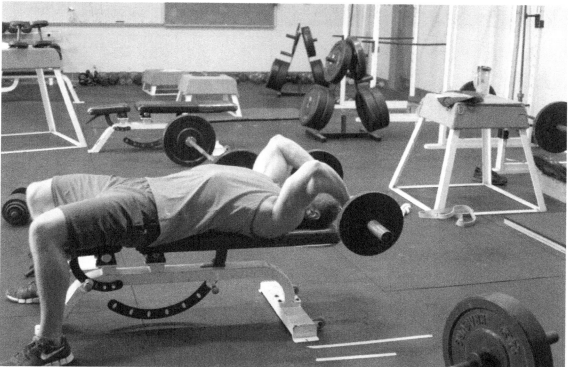

For seated and standing French presses, stand or sit with the weight directly overhead and lower it under control for a deep stretch. Be sure to keep your elbows somewhat pointing up – it is fine if the elbows jet out to the sides slightly, just make sure they don't angle laterally too much. Once in the bottom position, reverse the motion and extend your arms overhead once again.

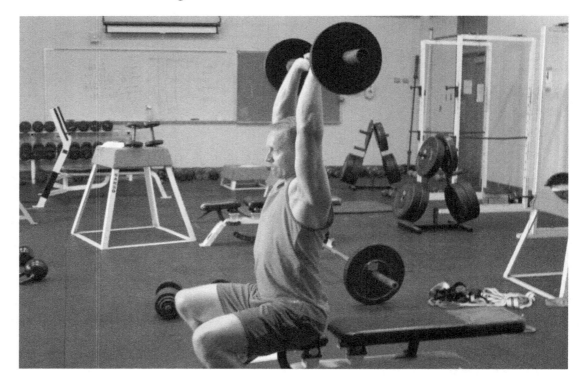

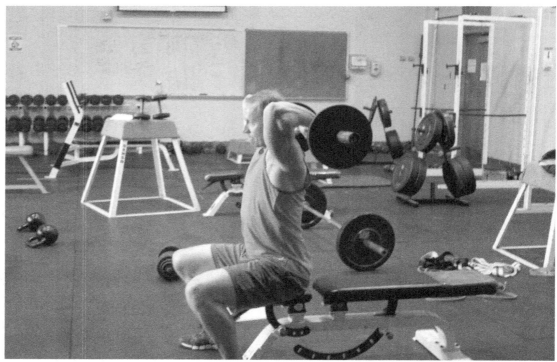

Tip: For a little variety in your skullcrushing efforts try performing the same movement on a decline or incline bench. Be sure to perform the movement the same as described above, however you may find yourself using slightly less weight on the decline bench and you will be able to use a little more weight on the incline bench.

Dumbbell and cable overhead extensions: Similar to the overhead French press, dumbbell and cable overhead extensions will treat the triceps to a deep growth-inducing stretch. Using a dumbbell or rope attachment may prove more comfortable for your elbows as they position the wrists and forearms in a more natural angle. For two-arm dumbbell extensions grasp a single dumbbell keeping both hands flat against the inside of the plates. With the weight directly overhead lower the weight behind your head feeling a deep stretch in your triceps and then return to the starting position.

You may also perform this movement single-arm with a lighter dumbbell. However, for the single-armed version, you will lower the dumbbell laterally instead of straight back. The elbow will be pointing outward and the dumbbell will travel behind your head for a deep stretch.

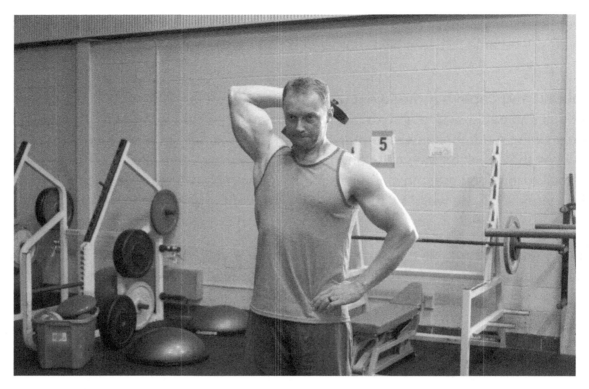

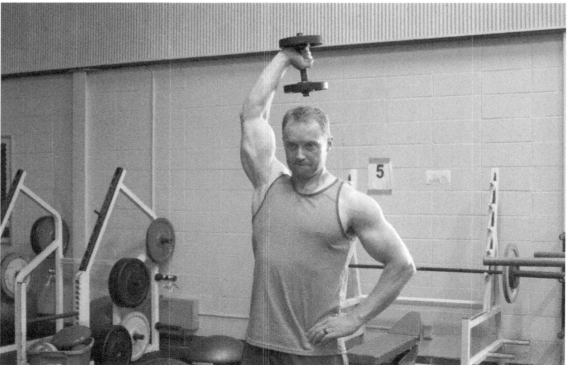

For overhead rope extensions, utilize similar form as described above. Grasp a rope attachment from a low pulley station and perform the movement in a rhythmic pattern making sure you use an appropriate amount of weight to complete the prescribed number of reps in a safe manner.

For a little variety rope extensions can also be performed horizontally by pulling from a pulley apparatus that is set about shoulder level and positioning your upper body parallel with the floor and in a slight lunge stance. Pulling the rope from behind your head, extend the cable perpendicular to the apparatus and squeeze the triceps.

Tip: Many gym-goers tend to set the cable apparatus pulley much too low for overhead rope extensions – this can sometimes create difficulty in getting into the correct position. A tip is to set the cable pulley about waist level to make it easier to get into that desired position. This will make it much less stressful on your back, shoulder, and other joints when starting and ending the movement.

Dips: Dips are an invaluable tool in the pursuit of bigger triceps. Not only are they effective in packing on the mass, they are also allow you to use a higher amount of resistance due to being a compound, multi-joint movement.

There are two types of dips being referred to. The first is the parallel dip. You may see many individuals utilize this move for chest development; however, it can be just as effective for triceps. Simply grasp the parallel bars that are about shoulder width with your arms straight - your body should be as perpendicular to the floor as possible. With your legs pointing somewhat straight below you, lower yourself while keeping your body as upright as possible and your elbows by your sides. This upright position will ensure the stress is placed on the triceps – if you lean too far forward and/or allow your arms to flare out to the sides, the stress is shifted to the chest. Lower yourself where you are comfortable and avoiding any shoulder pain. A good rule of thumb is to form a 90 degree angle in the elbow joint.

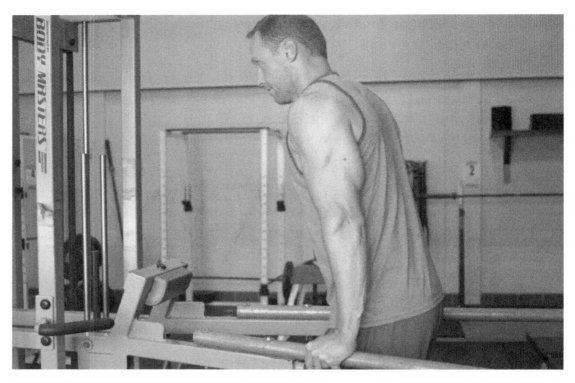

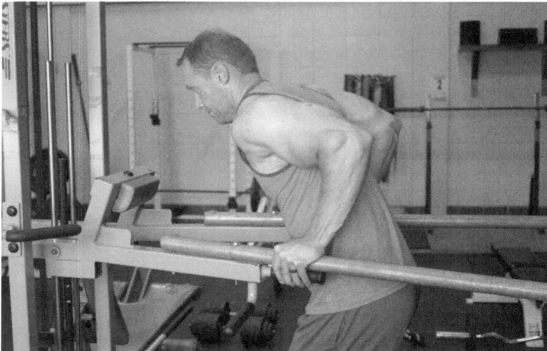

Be sure you can perform parallel dips for the desired reps and range of motion before utilizing a weight belt. Too many individuals try to lift too much weight and compromise their form and risk injury.

Another form of dips is the bench dip. This is performed with two benches side by side. Sit sideways on one bench grasping the edge of the bench on either side of your hips.

Place your feet on the other bench with just your heels touching and legs straight. Lift yourself off of the bench you are sitting on and drop your butt below the bench getting a 90 degree or so angle in your elbows. Extend back up to the top position straightening your arms and flexing your triceps then repeat.

Tip: A good way to really torch those tris once your strength has significantly improved on bench dips is to add a few plates to your lap. Once you have reached failure, have your workout partner take one plate off, then continue your set. Depending on how many plates you have to remove, continue this stripping method until you are doing your last set with just your bodyweight.

Close-grip bench press: Last but certainly not least is another compound favorite – the close-grip bench press. Again, since this is a multi-joint movement, more resistance is able to be placed on the triceps so be careful not to let your ego take over and lift too much weight or be unsafe in your technique. Lie back on a flat bench as if you were about to perform a bench press and grasp the bar with a shoulder width grip (any closer may put stress on your wrists). Un-rack the bar and lower the bar with your elbows close to your sides – this will ensure that most of the stress will be placed on the triceps and not the chest. Either you can touch the bar to your chest or an inch above it then return to the extended position. Flex your triceps hard at the top focusing on their contraction. Repeat making sure your elbows are not flaring out to the sides – keep them close to your body.

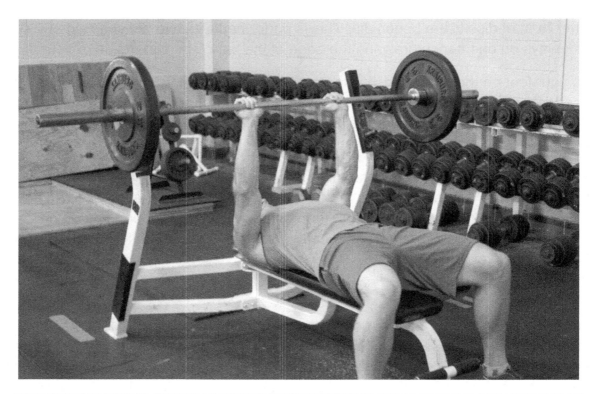

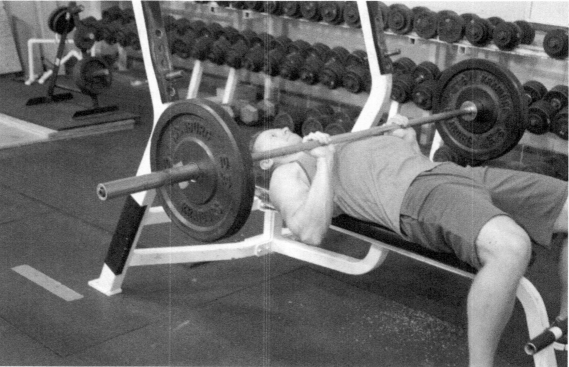

Tip: To put a new angle on an old favorite, try doing close-grip bench presses on a decline bench. This is somewhat similar to doing a pressdown with a free weight and will allow for a greater load on the bar. Performing these on a decline will also take a little stress off of the shoulder joints. Be sure to adhere to the same technique and safety concerns as described above.

The Biceps

Massive, well-peaked, muscular and separated biceps are the goal of so many. Hours upon hours of blood, sweat and tears go into training and torturing this often stubborn body part. We look up to our "brothers in arms" who have massive arms in hopes to find some kind of "secret" or magic program that we can put into practice. These guys have what we want; shapely, well-defined, huge biceps!

Who can blame us? When you hear, "make a muscle" we instantly think of our biceps. It is the quintessential beach muscle that instantly raises eyebrows when flexed to its extreme. Many in the power lifting arena see very little use for impressively built biceps, but in bodybuilding it is vital to a balanced and proportionate physique. Even if you never find yourself on the stage you still want to fill out those sleeves. What use is it to have a barrel chest and a wide back if your arms are tiny, little noodles?

One of the biggest mistakes made in gyms is overtraining and biceps are the most abused receiver. Some will toil for up to an hour at times performing set after set of barbell curls, dumbbell curls, and machine and cable curls in order to reach their goals. Many of these routines are put into practice without rhyme or reason – just a haphazard effort at best.

Programs are thrown together with blind faith and without much thought or strategy hoping that the muscle will develop. This chapter will define what it takes to build some impressive guns. Exercise selection, reps schemes, volume regulation, order of movements and rest intervals all have a profound effect on the outcome of your progress. So gulp down your protein shake and let's get busy!

Anatomy and function

Although the biceps may seem like a simple muscle to understand it is composed of two muscles that actually have dual functions (hence the name biceps).

Biceps brachii: This muscle makes up the major portion of the two muscles both originating in different places on the shoulder blade. The heads unite on the radius which has the ability to rotate. The main function of the biceps brachii is to flex the elbow and supinate (rotate out) the forearm. It is assisted by the brachialis and the brachioradialis (primarily a forearm muscle).

Brachialis: It originates near the middle of the front upper arm (known as the humerus). It connects at the top of the ulna just after it crosses the shoulder joint. Its main function is elbow flexion. Since it's connected to the ulna, which doesn't rotate, it's involved only in flexion of the elbow, not supination.

Biceps builders

Now that you know a little about anatomy and function, let's delve into what makes outstanding biceps. The movements presented are designed to get the most out of each trip to the gym. Remember to always use good form and not to use too much weight to compromise your safety.

Barbell and Dumbbell Curls: For overall biceps mass and strength nothing beats good ole fashion barbell and dumbbell curls. With a shoulder-width grip on barbell curls remember to keep your elbows by your sides and allow for a firm grip – don't squeeze the bar too hard as it will take away your focus from the biceps. Curl the bar up in a full range of motion and avoid resting the bar at the top of the movement. Curl up and squeeze hard then return to the starting position.

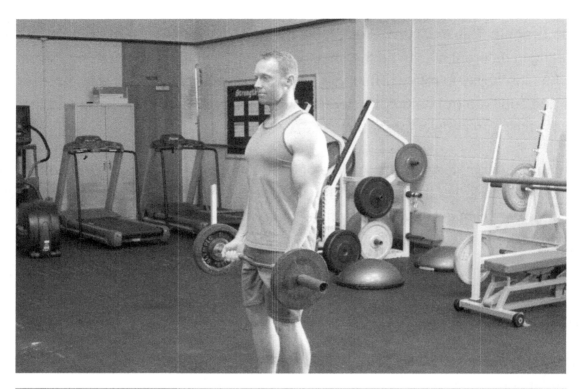

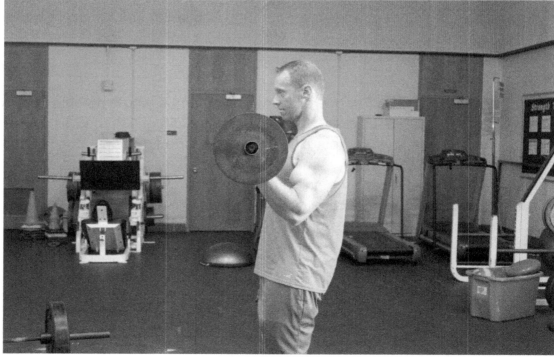

For dumbbell curls (which will additionally work the brachialis) start with the dumbbells by your side with your thumb side facing forward. Curl them up while simultaneously supinating your forearms – twisting until your thumbs are facing out at the top of the movement and your palms are facing up. Squeeze at the top and reverse the motion on the way down.

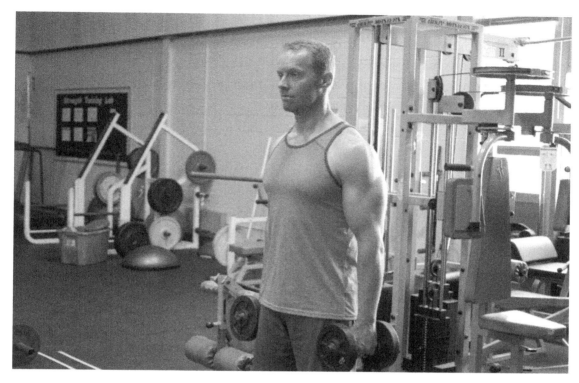

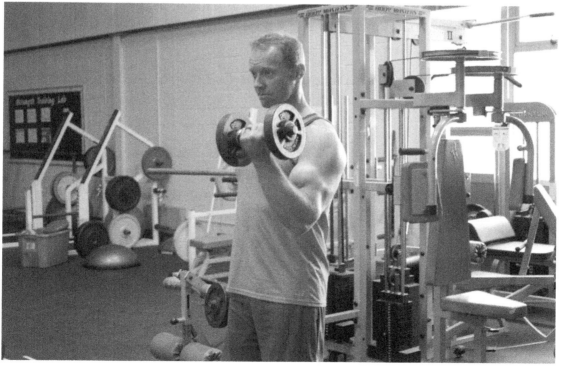

The standard cable curl (standing in front of a cable apparatus and mimicking a barbell curl) is a good way to mix up a routine. Due to its mechanics, the pulley action stresses the top portion of the movement for a more intense contraction.

Tip: Try different grips on the barbell curls to stress a different area of the muscle. For example: A narrow grip will build the outside portion of the biceps making them appear thicker from the front and a wide grip will stress the inside of the biceps making the front double biceps pose that much more impressive.

Barbell, EZ Bar and Dumbbell Preacher Curls: To really get at the lower biceps area preacher curls are a must. Be sure to use a full range of motion; all the way up to peak contraction and all the way down for a full extension. Pay close attention to the top portion of the movement – too many individuals like to rest the bar at the top. Avoid this. Instead, squeeze at the top without letting the tension decrease and immediately lower the weight. Try not to go too heavy as preacher curls can be a bit dangerous due to their strict nature. Also, if the straight bar tends to hurt your forearms try using the EZ bar for better wrist comfort.

For dumbbell preacher curls sit a little sideways on the bench for comfort as you perform this movement. Be sure to get an intense contraction at the top as with barbell preacher curls. The added bonus of the dumbbell version is that you are able to slightly twist the dumbbell with your pinky closer to your shoulder for a more intense contraction.

Many gyms are also equipped with a curl machine that mimics the barbell preacher curl. These are a great addition near the end of a routine when you want to "burn out" the biceps.

Tip: For an intense finisher to a biceps workout do this: After reaching failure on full range reps try doing partial pumps near the top third of the movement until you absolutely cannot move the weight. Your biceps will get be screaming for mercy!

Barbell and Dumbbell Spider Curls: Similar to preacher curls is the spider curl. Simply stand resting your chest on the pad where you would normally put your elbows. Your arms will be dangling straight down on the opposite side of the pad. Grab a barbell of light to moderate weight with a shoulder grip and curl up feeling an intense contraction. Return the weight until your arms are completely perpendicular to the floor. The advantage of spider curls as opposed to preacher curls is the constant tension especially at the top of the movement. Spider curls allow absolutely no rest when the bar is curled to the top.

With dumbbell spider curls perform them in the same fashion as dumbbell preacher curls. Remember to keep the tension on the muscle and try not to rest at the bottom of the motion. A light to moderate weight is all that is needed to get maximum benefit from this movement.

Tip: This is the perfect opportunity to put a new spin on an old trick – 21s! With a lighter weight than normal perform seven reps from the bottom to the half-way point, then perform seven reps from the mid-point to the top half of the motion, and finally do seven full range reps to finish off the set. Your biceps are guaranteed to be blitzed!

Incline Dumbbell Curls: As an old favorite of Arnold Schwarzenegger, incline dumbbell curls are unmatched at stretching out the biceps and creating a full muscle belly with peak. Adjust a weight bench to about 45 degrees (or a little higher if you are new to the movement). Lay back on the bench with your shoulders touching the pad (many make the mistake of leaning forward while doing these) and your arms straight down with dumbbells of moderate weight. Again, some of these movements are a bit isolated in nature so this is no time to throw around heavy weights and risk injury.

Start with your thumbs forward and supinate the dumbbells as you curl up as in standing dumbbell curls. Be sure to curl the weight along your sides and keep your shoulders on the pad. Come up to the top position and squeeze and then return to the starting position by reversing the motion.

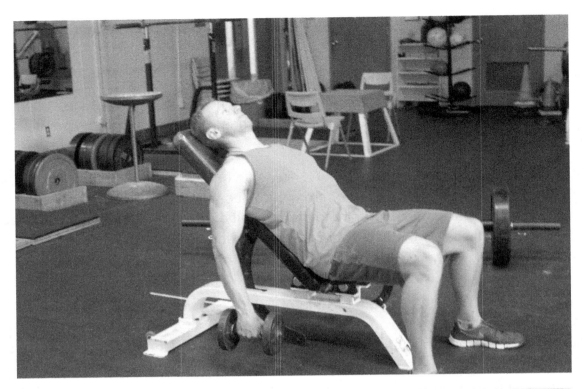

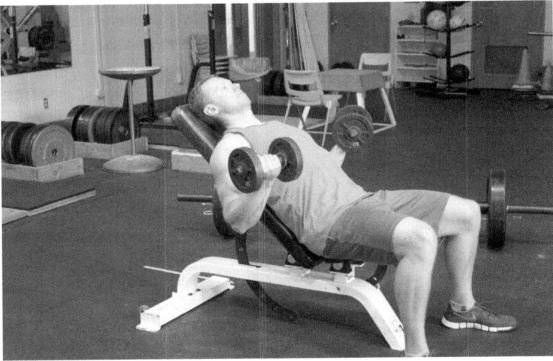

Tip: For an intense burn try doing incline curls with cables. Attach a "D" handle to a floor pulley and position the bench in front of the apparatus facing away. Curl with one arm then the other. The continuous tension will surely torch those biceps!

Concentration Curls: Normally reserved near the end of a biceps routine, concentration curls are a great movement when you need peak. Sit on the edge of a bench leaning over with a dumbbell and your elbow braced against your inner thigh. Curl the weight up to your shoulder and squeeze. Again, do not use a ton of weight. This is not the time to grab a big dumbbell and start swinging. Use a weight you can handle and control for moderate reps. Also, avoid heaving the weight up with your shoulder – it should be steady while the biceps is doing the work.

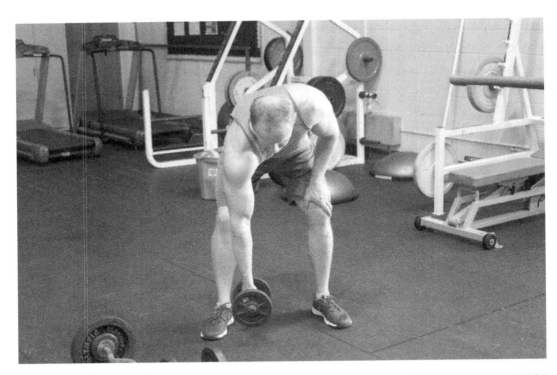

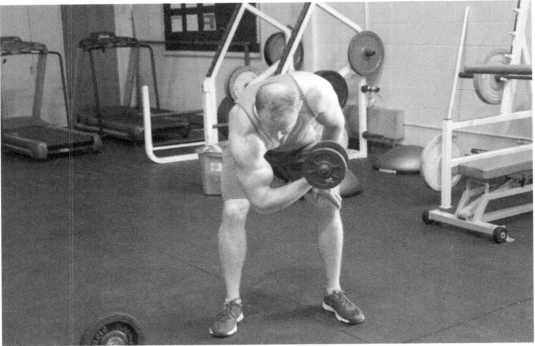

Tip: Although a bit more technical and with more skill involved you can alternately do standing concentration curls. Bend over at the waste holding a dumbbell straight down just a few inches off of the floor. Curl the weight up toward your shoulder while keeping your upper arm stationary. Resist bringing your elbow toward your body and keep it pointing straight down. Feel the biceps "knot up" at the top and then reverse the motion.

Hammer Curls: This dual functioning movement is great for both forearm mass and biceps peak. Hold the dumbbells with a thumb-forward grip by your sides. Without supinating the wrist, curl the weight up while keeping your wrist in a fixed position (this is the hammer motion). Curl up, squeeze and return. These can be performed either simultaneously or alternately.

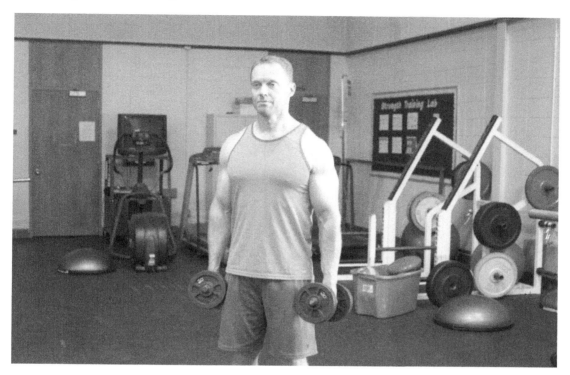

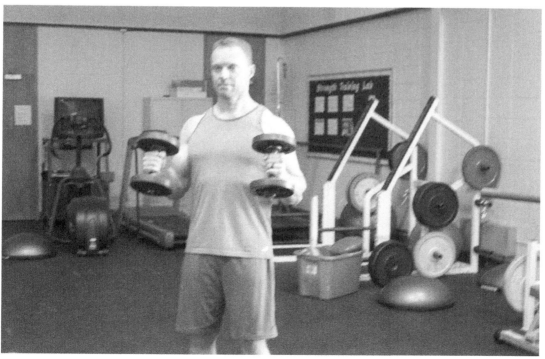

Tip: You may see many trainers do these with a slight variation. Begin in the same position, but as you curl the weight up move the dumbbell across your upper body toward your opposite shoulder keeping your upper arm stable. Alternate each side for all reps. Many claim a greater contraction and more comfort for the wrist area.

The Forearms

Many do not consider forearm training as a high priority item. Huge upper arms, a barrel chest, and thick quads are what most are after in any given gym in America – but what about the details? Sweating the small stuff is what completes a physique from head to toe. Hamstrings, calves, rear deltoids, and forearms are among those details that, when developed properly, can make all the difference toward a well-balanced and proportioned body.

Think of it, what are massive upper arms without a pair of well-built forearms to go with them? Not only will they complement your look, you will also develop strength and function to facilitate other lifts and subsequently help you pack on mass in other areas such as back, shoulders, and biceps.

Now, forearms do get some stimulation from other lifts such as curls, rows, and pull-ups/pulldowns, but in order for you to fully reach your forearm potential (especially if it happens to be a weak point) you must add in some specialized training to your program. This is not to say that a movement or two should just be thrown into the end of an arm day haphazardly performed with minimal intensity. Forearm training deserves every bit of focus and discipline as a set of squats or bench presses. A well thought-out plan of action including proper volume, intensity, and the use of a variety of angles is the best way to ensure maximum development is achieved.

Anatomy and function

The forearm is surprisingly a complex group of small muscle groups with several functions. The **brachialis** and **brachioradialis** both contribute to elbow flexion and aid the forearm while curling, which are worked during many curl motions. The **pronator teres** aids the forearm in pronation as well as elbow flexion. The flexors (**palmaris longus, flexor carpi radialis**, and **flexor carpi ulnaris**) curl the palm in while the extensors (**extensor carpi ulnaris** and **extensor carpi radialis brevis**) flex the palm out. A comprehensive resistance training program should include movements for all areas of the forearm in order for complete development.

Forearm builders

Now that you know a little about anatomy and function, let's delve into what makes outstanding forearms. The movements presented are designed to get the most out of each trip to the gym. Remember to always use good form and not to use too much weight to compromise your safety.

Wrist curls: The basic wrist curl (working more of the flexors) can be performed either with a barbell, cable, or a pair of dumbbells. The advantage of utilizing dumbbells is when you have limited rotation of the forearms and find it difficult to use a straight bar. Simply grab the weight at about shoulder width and either lay your forearms across a bench or on your thighs where our hands can extend down toward the floor. Begin by stretching out your forearms and letting the weight lower toward the floor while keeping a firm grip on the bar. Reverse the motion and return to the top for a strong contraction. This will be a short range of motion so try to avoid bouncing or jerking the weight during the movement as injury may occur.

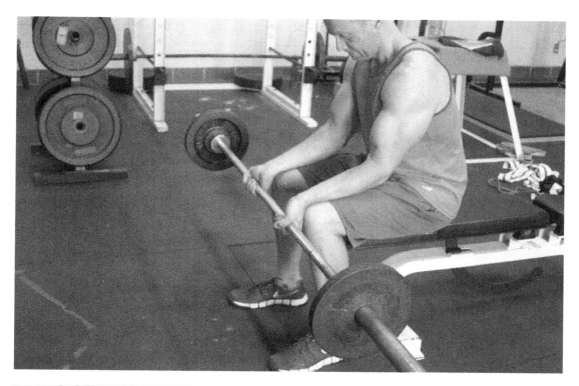

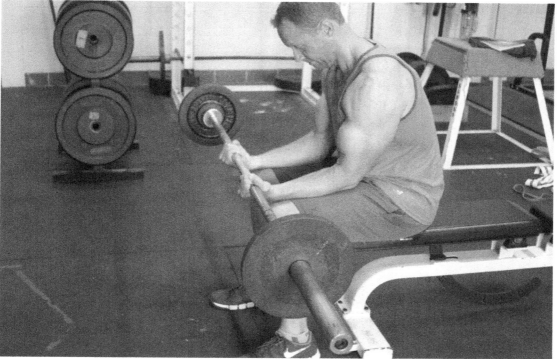

Tip: For those who find that placing your forearms over a bench or your knees is a bit too uncomfortable, try behind-the-back wrist curls. Stand while holding a barbell with an overhand grip behind your thighs. With your forearms against your glutes for support, using only your hands, curl the barbell up for a contraction. Performing the movement this way can sometimes alleviate the pain some may have in the stretch position of a traditional wrist curl.

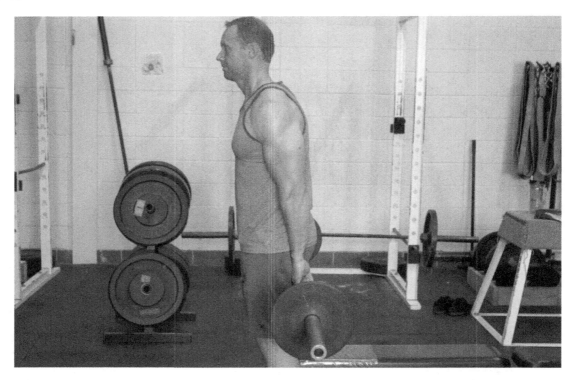

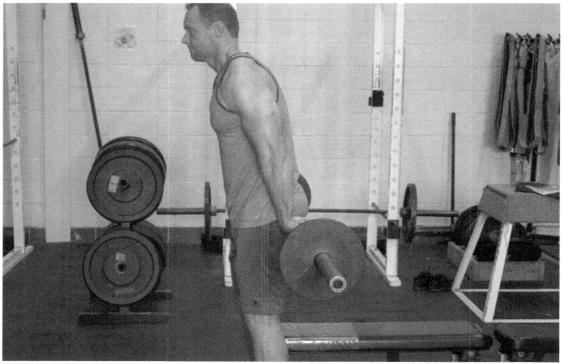

Reverse wrist curls: Much like the wrist curl, the reverse wrist curl is performed in a similar fashion only with your palms facing down working your extensors. Hold a barbell, cable handle or a set of dumbbells over a bench or your thighs with your palms facing the floor, let the weight stretch your extensors then reverse the motion for a contraction to the top. Remember to control the movement and avoid swinging the weight.

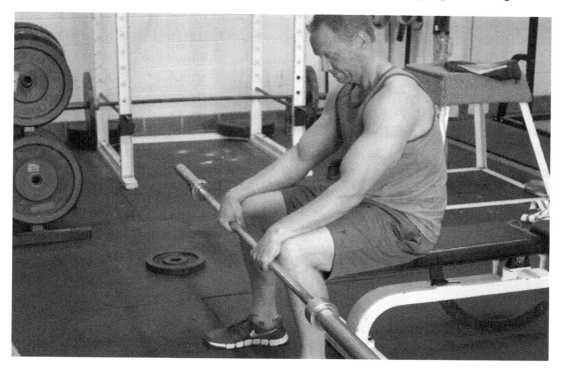

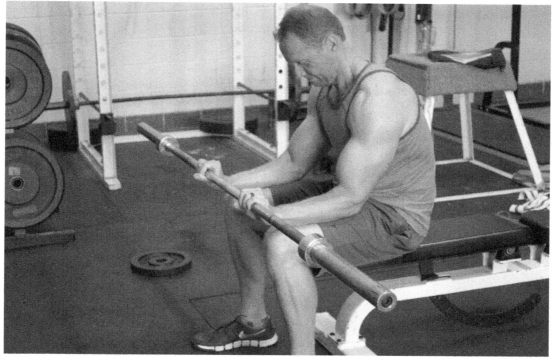

Tip: For an intense rep try holding each contraction for a few seconds at the top. You will not have to use much weight at all, but the burn will be worth it!

Hammer curls: Normally reserved for a biceps workout, hammer curls are a great addition to a complete forearm program. Working the brachialis and brachioradialis along with the biceps, hammer curls will also help develop peak in the biceps. Simply hold a pair of dumbbells by your sides with your thumbs facing forward. Without supinating the forearm, curl the weight up toward your shoulder – this should look like a hammering motion. Return to your side and repeat.

Tip: Another way to perform (and some find it more effective) is cross-body hammer curls. Perform the movement as described above, but instead of curling by your side you will curl the dumbbell across your upper body toward your opposite shoulder. Alternate each arm.

Reverse curls: Another great alternative to hammer curls are reverse barbell curls. Perform a barbell curl as you would during a biceps workout, but reverse your grip on the bar at about shoulder width. Be sure to keep strict form and choose a moderate weight.

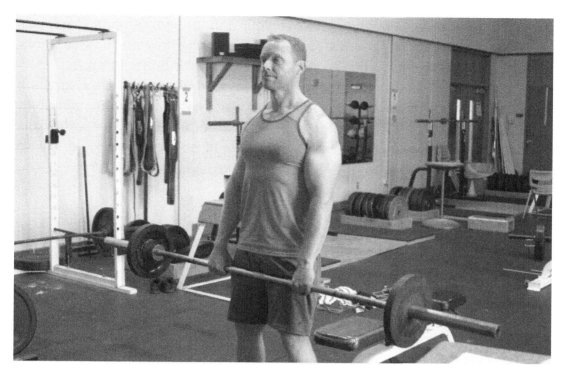

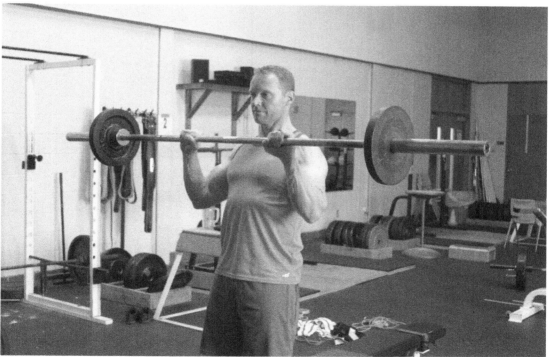

Tip: For the ultimate in isolated forearm training try performing reverse curls on a preacher bench. This will not only prevent any cheating of the movement, it will also ensure isolation of the muscles being trained. Again, choose a moderate weight as these can be very difficult to perform with a significant amount of weight.

Grip Work: There are many ways to improve your grip for strength and mass in the forearms. Exercise grips, the absence of using straps on certain back movements, and gripping weight plates are just a few techniques to utilize for better forearm development. One effective and convenient technique to utilize is to firmly grip the bar at the end of all wrist curl sets. For example, after each set of wrist curls curl up the weight in the contracted position and squeeze the bar for five to ten seconds. This will be difficult after your normal set, but will improve grip strength and add intensity to your forearm program.

The Quadriceps

Mighty, well-built quadriceps is a true sign of utter power on a physique. Huge, thickly developed, sweeping quads can differentiate you from the rest of the pack. It can make all the difference between a balanced, well-proportioned aesthetically pleasing physique and a top–heavy, stick-legged candy apple body.

Now, we can't all possess professional bodybuilder-sized quads, but we can develop big, thick, well proportioned, and separated quad muscles that would be impressive by any standard. Don't get caught years from now wishing you had trained your quads a little harder or dedicated more time to them. I cannot tell you how many times I see individuals in gyms workout with pants on in the dead heat of summer just to hide their lack of dedication and development regarding quad training.

The quadriceps make up a huge amount of muscle mass on our bodies. They are challenging to train, with countless hours in the gym and gallons of sweat required for what seems to be just a few ounces of muscle. Training quads intensely will give the entire body an opportunity to grow due to the natural growth hormone and testosterone surge you will initiate.

A squat, for example, requires a huge amount of muscle from the entire body in order to drive the weight up – quads, hams, back, traps, shoulders, and abs all contribute to move and/or stabilize the weight during the lift. This will only spell growth that surges throughout the body constructing one powerful-looking build. You have to ask yourself one question: Do I want that?

Anatomy and function

The quadriceps is a large muscle group that comprises of four main muscles on the front of the thigh. Let's take a quick look at what comprises the muscles of the quadriceps and their function.

Rectus femoris: Originating from the ilium, the rectus femoris occupies the middle of the thigh covering most of the other three quadriceps muscles.

Vastus lateralis: Originating from the femur, the vastus lateralis extends down the lateral side (outer area) of the thigh and inserts into the patella.

Vastus medialis: Also originating from the femur, the vastus medialis extends down the medial side (inner area) of the thigh and inserts into the patella. This muscle makes up the much sought-after "tear drop" look.

Vastus intermedius: This muscle lies between the vastus lateralis and vastus medialis on the front of the femur inserting into the patella.

All four quadriceps muscles extend the knee joint. Additionally, the rectus femoris, due to its originating location, also flexes the hip joint.

Quad builders

Now that you know a little about anatomy and function, let's delve into what makes outstanding quadriceps. The movements presented are designed to get the most out of each trip to the gym. Remember to always use good form and not to use too much weight to compromise your safety.

Back squats: The back squat (the so called granddaddy of leg movements) is the quintessential exercise for developing impressive quads. Get under the bar in a squat rack and place the bar on a comfortable position across your upper back on your trapezius muscle. Grasp the bar with both hands out to the sides on the bar for stability. Now, step back from the rack into a shoulder-width stance or a little wider.

This is crucial: begin the movement by bending your knees first. Do not bend at the hips or back at the beginning of the movement, this will cause you to pitch forward. Lower the weight until your hamstrings touch your calves or you reach a comfortable range of motion (ROM). Drive the weight back up first utilizing your hips and then your knees. Do not lock your legs out at the top.

Important note: the range of motion is entirely up to the individual. Using a full ROM is always the most ideal way to perform any exercise, but squats can raise questions regarding knee pain and back strain. For a rule of thumb, descend as far as you are comfortable and then return to the start. Just remember not to short change yourself and take it as a challenge. Squats are a tough movement, but the reward is well worth it.

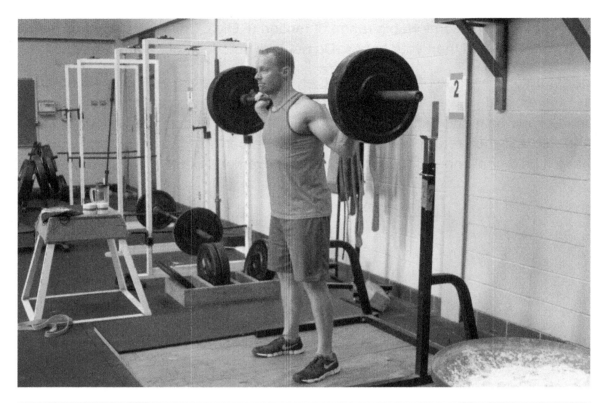

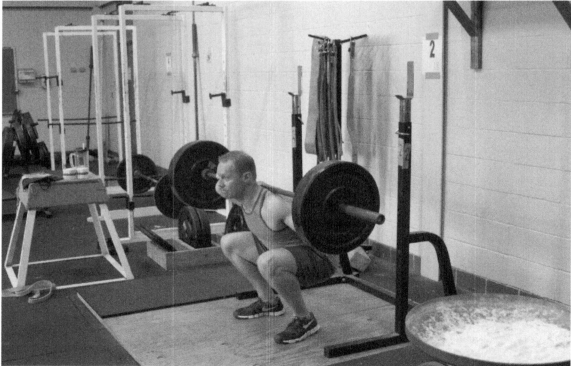

Tip: Be sure that your knees stay in-line with your toes. Do not allow your knees to cave in or bow out too far. Keeping them in-line will ensure healthy knees and more generation of strength.

Front squats: For front squats position yourself under the bar in front of you and rest the bar in the crook of your shoulder girdle across your deltoids. Cross your forearms over one another and steady the bar on either side. Keep your upper arms parallel with the floor and your head up. Pick up the weight and step back with a shoulder-width stance. Perform the movement as you would a back squat. You will notice that you are able to keep your back a little straighter throughout this movement. Front squats target the quads a little better than the traditional back squat which involves more hip, hams and glutes strength.

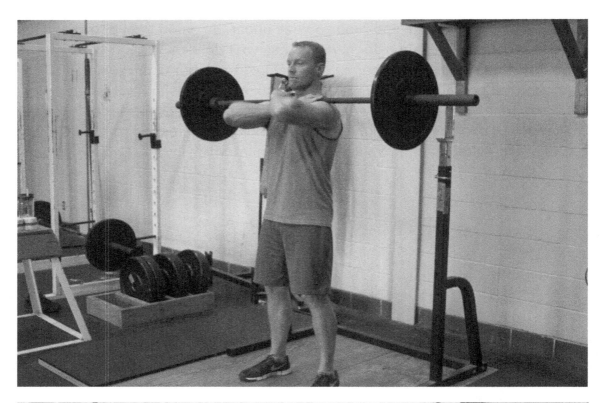

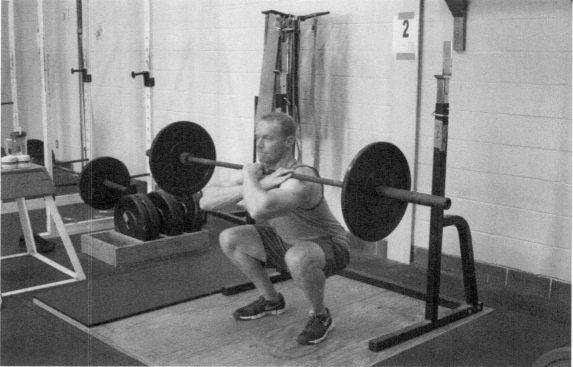

Tip: If you are new to front squats and need added stability, perform them on a Smith machine for a while until you are comfortable with handling the weight.

Tip: If you are a tall trainer and find yourself either pitching too far forward or your heels are rising off of the floor at the bottom of the movement, try placing a five or ten pound plate under each heel for added stability. This can be applied to either squat variation.

Hack squats: To focus a little more on the outer sweep (vastus lateralis) of the quad nothing beats the hack squat. With a moderate weight place yourself comfortably under the pads of the machine and take a shoulder width stance in the middle of the foot plate. Descend until you reach a full ROM and then return to the starting position. Make sure not to accelerate into the descent too much as this will put too much strain on your knees. Keep the movement at a steady pace. Again, as with most leg movements, do not lock out your knees at the top.

Tip: Some gyms are not equipped with a hack squat machine, but do not despair, there is a solution. Simply grasp a loaded barbell from behind your calves (kind of a deadlift but with the weight behind your legs). With your back straight and your head up, begin lifting with your legs until you are almost standing straight up. Without locking your legs return the weight to the starting position without touching the floor. This movement requires very strict form and a moderate weight that can be handled easily until you are comfortable.

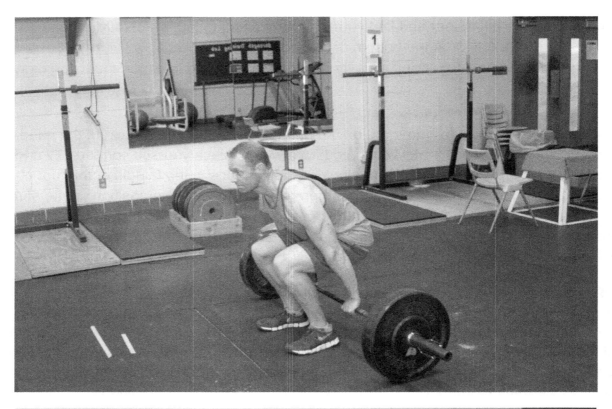

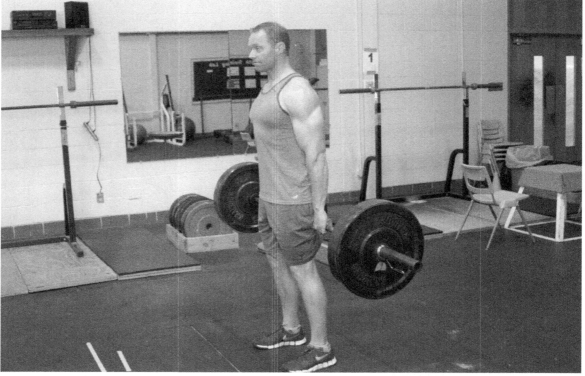

Leg press: Another great mass builder is the traditional 45 degree angled leg press. The advantage of this machine is that it places very little if any stress on the lumbar area and focuses on the thighs to a greater extent. Seat yourself in the machine and make sure the seat is back far enough for a full ROM. Place your feet about shoulder width apart in the middle of the foot plate. Push up the weight without locking your knees and turn down the safety catches. Lower the weight under control and explode back up to the starting position. Go as far down as you can with the weight before your lower back starts to round. Also, try to avoid half or partial reps – you are just cheating yourself out of developing your quads to the fullest.

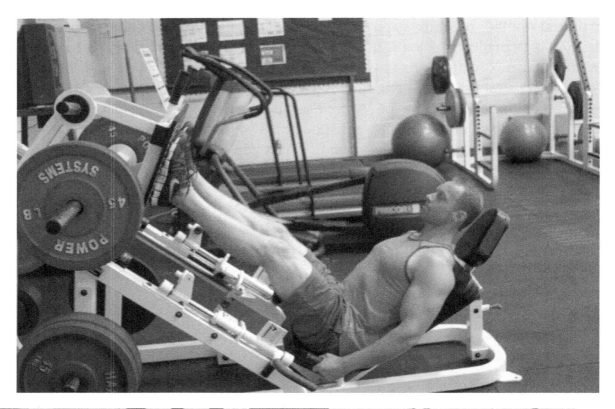

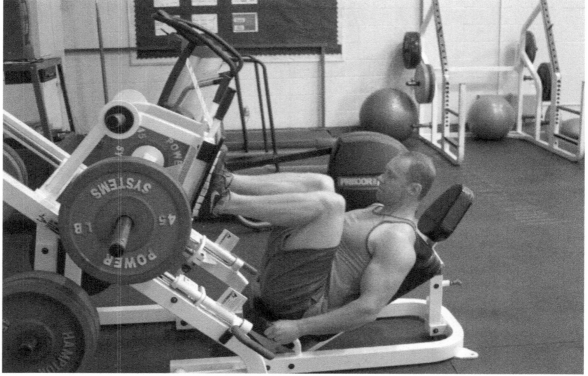

Tip: If you find the leg press in your gym to constantly be occupied or your gym simply does not have this piece of equipment there are other options to choose from. Many gyms have alternate machine leg presses to utilize including weight selectorized versions as well as Hammer Strength brand.

Leg extensions: For ultimate isolation of the quad muscles nothing comes close to the leg extension machine. Sit into the machine with your knees lined up with the axle of the action arm and your back flat against the back pad. Adjust the shin pad so it fits right into the 90 degree angle of your foot and ankle. Lift the weight at a moderate pace and squeeze at the top without pause, then return to the start. Try to avoid holding the weight up at the top and doing too much weight as this may put unnecessary stress on your knees, specifically the patella tendon.

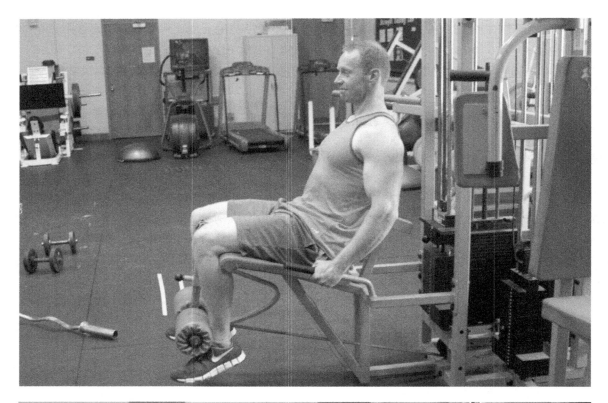

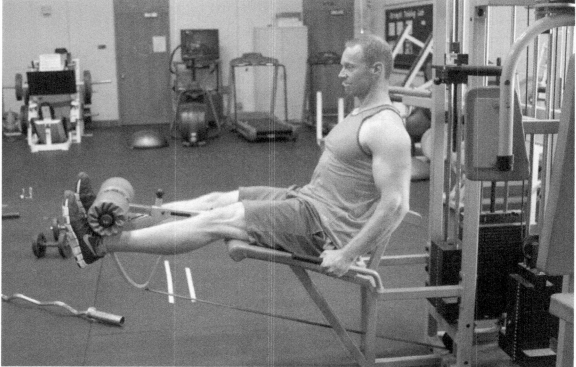

Tip: For a bit of a shock to the top portion of your quads and a wicked burn try this variation of the leg extension. Perform the movement as described above, but this time lean your upper body forward off of the back pad so you are 90 degrees or less to your legs in the top position. You will have to lighten the weight a bit, but the reward will be one intense burn!

Lunges: Lunges are a great shape movement for the quads. They give your thighs that nice round look and really tie each muscle in together. While some may profess that lunges are a total thigh exercise with an equal amount of ham and glute involvement, for the sake of this chapter we will focus on how lunges can be applied specifically to quad training.

Place a relatively light barbell across your shoulders as you would on back squats. Step back from the squat rack and step forward with one leg well in front of you. Bend down on that leg so that your knee is just a few inched from the floor. You want to avoid striking your knee to the floor. Also, make sure your knee does not travel over your toes – if they are, step out further. You trailing foot will stay back the entire time. Once you are in the down position power yourself up into the upright starting position and bring your lunging foot back next to your trailing foot. Repeat with the opposite leg – this will count as one rep.

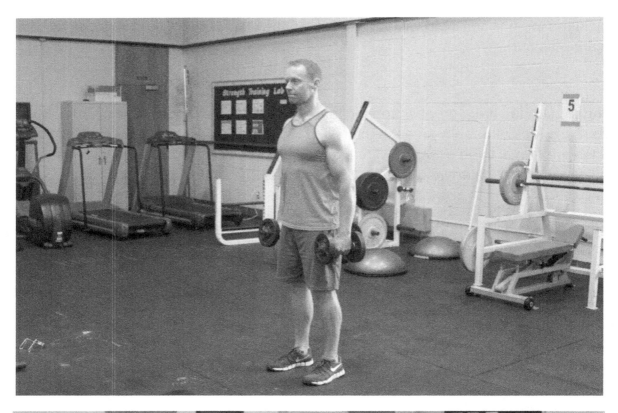

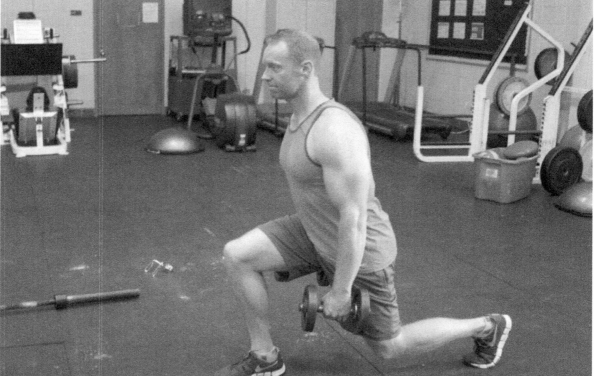

Tip: A great alternative to barbell lunges is the Smith machine lunge. Simply start with one leg in the lunge position and complete all reps with that leg. You will not return to the start after each rep, you will stay forward, complete all reps for that leg and then switch legs and repeat.

Tip: Another favorite is the walking lunge. These are performed in a spacious area of your gym and make sure you have at least 30 or so feet of "runway" space to walk. Walking lunges are just that – you will lunge forward and then walk the trailing leg forward to meet the other foot in the starting position and lunge again with the opposite leg. It is a constant walking motion.

The Hamstrings

Balance is not only a principle when it comes to aesthetics and proportions for your physique; it also plays a pivotal role in the practical functionality of performance in and out of the gym. Certain antagonistic muscles are crucial for the strength, muscle mass development and performance of their counterparts, therefore specific focus and balance of other factors such as volume and intensity are a must for any athlete.

Enter hamstrings. No one sees them, no one ever tells you to flex them, why spend so much thought, time and effort into improving them? Why? The athletes who did their homework on every single aspect of preparation pertaining to development, conditioning, and balance are the ones victorious in the end. Hamstrings should be no different when it comes to a complete physique.

Sure, your quads steal the spotlight regarding attention in and out of the gym but now it is time to focus on its favorite relative; the hamstrings. Although sometimes difficult to develop, once built, hamstrings can become a serious strength that will support the quads, increase strength for other lifts and bring overall balance to your physique. So let's look at the hamstring complex a little closer and get ready to beef up the backs of those legs!

Anatomy and function

The hamstrings are a group of muscles comprised of three main muscles on the back of the thigh. Let's take a quick look at what comprises the main muscles of the hamstrings and their function.

Biceps femoris (located along the outside of the thigh), **semitendinosus** (located in the middle), and the **semimembranosus** (located on near the inside of the thigh) all originate just underneath the gluteus maximus on the pelvic bone and attach on the tibia of the lower leg. The functions of the hamstrings are knee flexion (bringing the heel towards the buttocks), hip extension (moving the leg to the rear), and deceleration of the lower leg.

When speaking of function it is easy to grasp the importance of hamstring development as it relates to other muscle movement performance. For instance, hamstrings play a vital role in the function of the squat, hack squat, front squat, leg press and lunge motions. Balance, therefore, is not only a visual aspect worth value on stage or the beach, but also as important while training the entire lower body. Without properly trained hamstrings, the quadriceps will not be able to be trained to their full potential.

Hamstring builders

Now that you know a little about anatomy and function, let's delve into what makes outstanding hamstrings. The movements presented are designed to get the most out of each trip to the gym. Remember to always use good form and not to use too much weight to compromise your safety.

Lying leg curl and seated leg curl: As an old standard, the lying leg curl machine is an extremely effective tool for hamstring isolation particularly the lower portion. Simply adjust the foot pad so it will rest on the back of the Achilles tendon. Your knees should be aligned with the axle of the machine for proper movement. Place your feet at approximately shoulder width on the pad. Next, curl up until the pad is near or touching the backs of your legs or buttocks then return to the starting position under control straightening your legs but not letting the weight stack hit at the bottom.

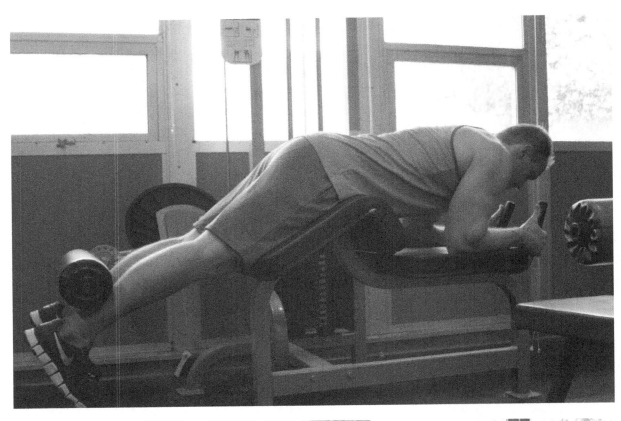

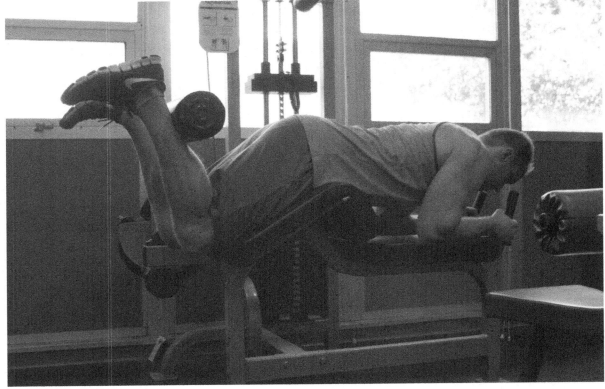

For the seated leg curl it should be a similar set-up. Adjust the pad as above and adjust the seat so your knee again aligns with the axle of the machine. Secure the top pad firmly against your thighs so you are locked into the machine. Perform the movement in a controlled motion curling under your thighs until you feel a strong contraction. Avoid partial movement so be sure to use a moderate amount of weight to allow for a full range of motion.

Tip: Try varying your foot/lower leg positions on the pads to hit different parts of your hams. For example: do a set with a wide stance, another with a shoulder width, and the last with the legs close together. This will ensure you are hitting each part of the hamstring for more balanced development.

Standing (one legged) leg curl: Similar to the lying and seated varieties, the standing leg curl machine gives you the opportunity to isolate one leg at a time. Training in this unilateral way also helps contract the muscle harder with each rep as it reaches the peak of the movement. Simply situate yourself into the machine (most have you place one knee on a pad and the other behind the ankle pad). Curl up the working leg for a full range of motion and contract the hamstring hard. It is easy to twist the lower body to cheat a few more reps out, but try to avoid this. This not only will cheat you out of proper development, but will also put you at risk for injury to the lower back/trunk area. Return the weight to the start position without letting the weight stack rest. Be sure to keep continuous tension on the muscle being worked at all times.

Tip: When performing a unilateral movement such as standing leg curls try your best to alternate legs without much rest. When one leg is working, the other is resting, therefore there is no reason to take a break after each set; a few seconds are fine, but try to avoid a normal rest period. Your hams will thank you!

Romanian deadlift and stiff-legged deadlift: A common confusion within the resistance training world is the difference between the Romanian deadlift (RDL) and the stiff-legged deadlift (SLDL). First, the RDL is performed with slightly bent knees and the weight hanging straight down. This movement is mainly to target the hamstring and glute muscles. The SLDL is performed with mostly straight legs (some lock out their knees) and a slightly rounded lower back. This movement is utilized to target the hamstrings and lower back. Both exercises have merit regarding hamstring development. Unlike the leg curl machines, the RDL and SLDL will put more stress on the glute and upper hamstring tie-in area.

For RDLs position a barbell in front of you and take a shoulder width stance. Grasp the barbell with a shoulder width grip and deadlift it up to the start position (it should be against your thighs). Put a slight bend in your knees and lock into this position (your knees should remain in this semi-bent angle throughout the movement). Rotating from the hips – NOT THE BACK – lower the barbell to about mid-shin level feeling your hamstrings stretch. Without jerking the weight, reverse the direction and come up to upper thigh level without coming up straight – this will keep the tension on the hams. Remember to rotate from the hips and keep your back as straight as possible which will feel like you are sticking your butt out behind you. Use a light weight at first to get the form down, then once you master the movement you can start adding weight.

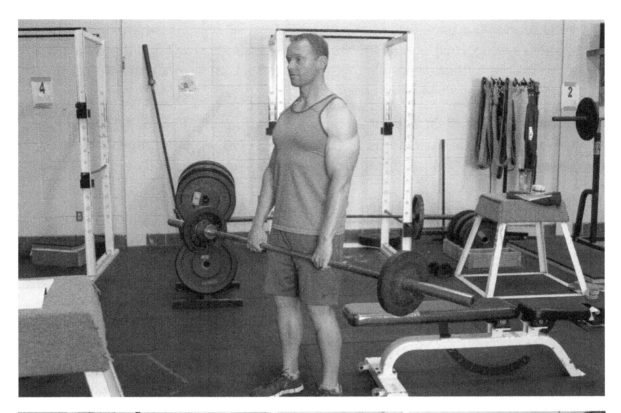

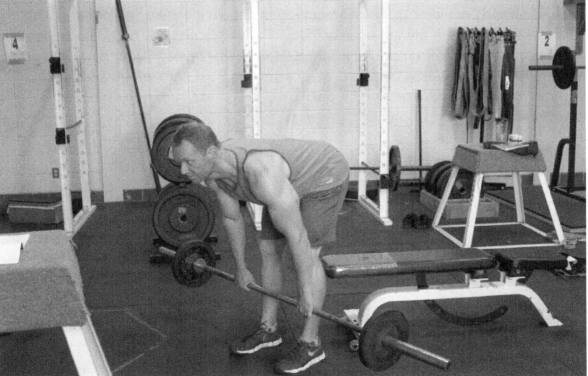

For SLDLs position your feet and hands as with the RDLs. This time with your knees locked (or almost locked) lower the bar down while letting your back round slightly. DO

NOT overly round your back with heavy weight! This will only cause an injury. The bar should travel close to your legs as the weight descends. You will find that you are able to lower the weight further using this method so use a light to moderate weight and perform the movement slowly and under control.

So which is it? RDL or SLDL? For the beginner stick to perfecting the RDL, but for the seasoned lifter, try throwing in some SLDLs once every third or fourth workout to change things up a bit. You will have to use a lighter weight, but the deep stretch will quickly make up for it.

Tip: A good alternative to is to use dumbbells instead of barbells. Dumbbells allow the ability to adjust your form slightly and are convenient in a crowded gym when a barbell station is hard to come by. Try both versions and see what works best for you.

Glute/ham raise: An old movement that has had a resurgence of popularity recently (for good reason) is the glute/ham raise. This particular movement requires a great deal of strength from the hamstrings and not too many individuals are able to initially do these correctly. Position yourself face down on a hyperextension bench with your heels under the foot pads and your knees on the hip pad. Situate yourself so that your knees will be the rotating point for this movement – you should look like you are kneeling on the bench. Starting from the top position, slowly lower your upper body – only bending at the knees – until you are parallel with the floor. In this position your body should form a straight line. Then reverse the direction contracting your hamstrings and "leg curl" your upper body back into the upright position.

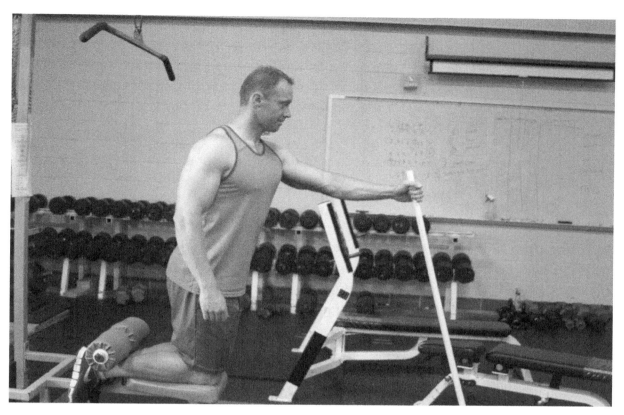

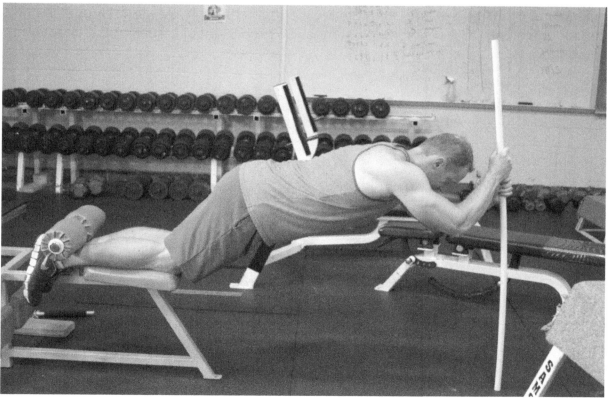

Tip: This is a tough movement so you may only get a few reps if any. A trick to get you going early on would be to use a small bar to help you with the upward motion. Simply grasp a small bar and place the other end on the floor – the bar should be perpendicular to the floor. Use the bar much like a hiker's pole and help your upper body up into the upright position. Once you master the movement and gain ample strength, you can get rid of the "crutch" and get to work!

Tip: Another remedy would be to start by using a hyperextension bench that is angled (about 45 degrees). This will allow you to perform more reps and master your form.

Leg press (feet high on plate): The name says it all. Once you have exhausted your hamstring on some of the isolation movements, leg presses with a high stance on the foot plate can be a very effective ham builder. Be sure to place them high enough to push through with your heels so that you feel a nice stretch in the bottom position.

Tip: Try wide and close stances with your feet to work all areas of the hamstrings.

Lunge: Traditionally utilized as a quad finishing movement, the lunge can be vital in creating that great side quad/ham tie-in look. Lunges not only work and stretch the quads, but also equally work the hamstrings. See more about lunges in the chapter on quadriceps.

The Calves

We all have a love/hate relationship with the "G" word: Genetics. When we are genetically gifted in certain areas of our physique we deem ourselves blessed. But, when we confront difficulty and monumental challenges we curse our genetics and all but give up on ourselves in attaining that coveted symmetrical and proportioned body we strive for each and every day. How is it that we excel in building some body parts but not others?

In all of my years training, I have come across maybe only a handful of individuals who were satisfied with their calf size. Others are at their wits end regarding trying to pack on reasonable amounts of muscle tissue to their lower legs and have relegated there training to just a few sets at the end of a leg day.

I am hoping the following will shed a little light and hope for those out there still yearning to build some impressive lower legs. You may not be able to build huge, striated bowling balls, but I honestly do believe most anyone can add a significant amount of muscle to their calves and improve the overall proportion of their physique. You DO like to wear shorts in the summer… right?

To pack on a significant amount of muscle on a weak point is a pretty heady task. It will take focus, determination, discipline and attention to detail. To manipulate such a weak area (no matter what body part it is) will take adjustments in frequency, volume and technique. Throwing in a few sets of calf raises at the end of a brutal quad and hamstring workout has not and will not do the trick. What you need is an overhaul in regard to training AND mentality. Having the belief that you can achieve that goal is imperative to your success. Without that belief, you will go nowhere, fast.

Treat the techniques below as you would an intense series of bench presses or squats. Full range of motion, stretching and squeezing the muscle will set you on the right path to results over a period of time. Have patience, be persistent and let's get to it!

Anatomy and function

The musculature of the lower leg is comprised of three main muscle groups. Let's take a look at each and there functions.

Gastrocnemius: This calf muscle which has two heads (medial and lateral) originates behind the knee on the femur and attaches to the heel with the Achilles tendon. These heads form the famous diamond shape everyone is looking to build and is mostly targeted when the knees are straight during movements.

Soleus: This muscle lies underneath the Gastrocnemius on the rear of the lower leg. It is mostly activated while the knees are bent.

Tibialis Anterior: This much neglected muscle is found on the front of the lower leg and is responsible for dorsi flexion of the foot (pointing the foot up). The importance of the tibialis anterior is that it aids in the balance of the lower leg regarding strength, muscle mass and injury prevention.

Calf builders

Now that you know a little about anatomy and function, let's delve into what makes outstanding calves. The movements presented are designed to get the most out of each trip to the gym. Remember to always use good form and not to use too much weight to compromise your safety.

Standing calf raises: This movement is the time-tested standard for building overall calf mass, particularly the gastrocnemius area. To perform this movement, fix your shoulders underneath the pads of the machine and stand with the balls of your feet on the calf block below about shoulder width apart. Stand with straight legs and just a slight bend in the knees to relieve the tension on that joint.

The knees should stay in this semi-locked position throughout the motion. Descend by lowering your heels toward the ground slowly. Once you have reached full range of motion and feel a deep stretch in the calves, reverse the motion and come up on the balls of your feet and contract the muscle as much as possible.

Important note: When coming up on the balls of your feet, do not try to flex your toes – let the foot do the movement. Also, DO NOT bounce the weight at the bottom or do a bouncing motion throughout the movement. So many individuals perform calf raises this way and benefit very little from their efforts. Full extension and full contraction at a steady, controlled pace is the way to go for real results.

Tip: If your gym does not have a normal selectorized standing calf raise machine there is an alternative. Try doing Smith machine standing calf raises. Affix a calf block under a loaded bar and perform calf raises as described above. No block? Try free weight plates or group exercise steps.

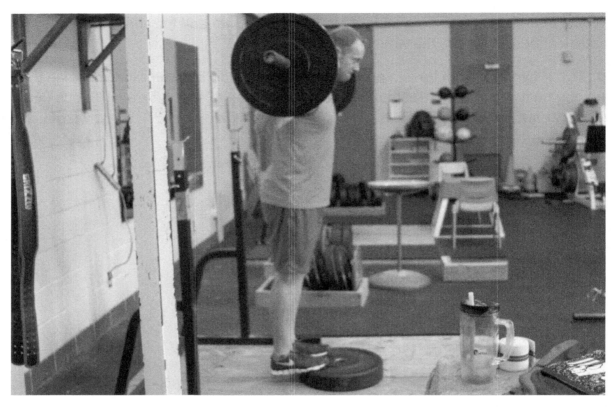

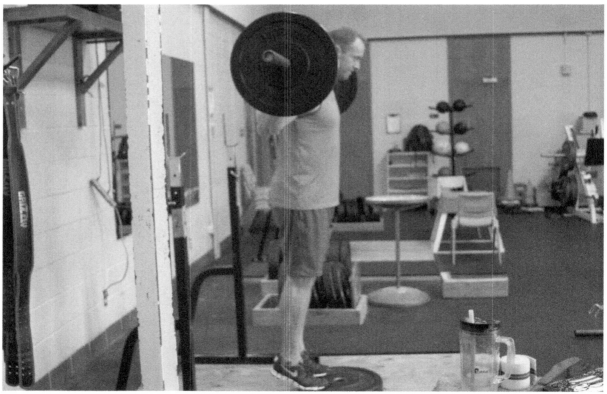

Seated calf raises: Another great standard in any calf program is the seated calf raise targeting the soleus muscle. This movement is great at adding width to the calf when seen from the front and thickness when viewed from the side. Fix your knees, not your thighs, under the pads of the machine and place your feet on the foot platform below at about shoulder width. As with the standing version, utilize a full range of motion – feel the stretch and then flex the calf hard at the top. Again, no bouncing!

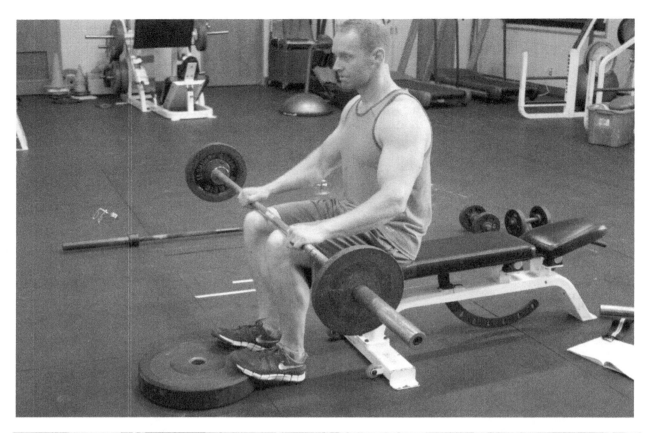

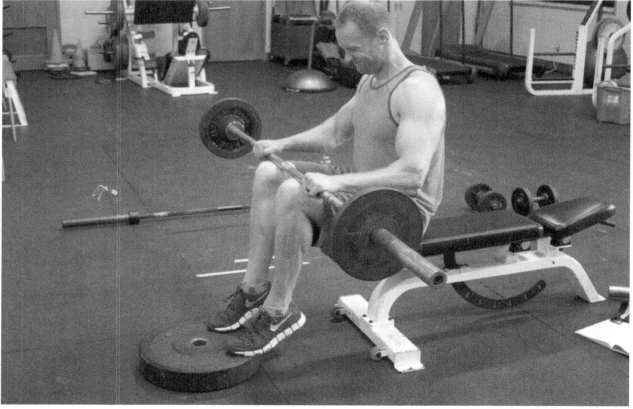

Tip: If you find yourself in a gym without a seated calf raise machine try rigging one of your own. You can either use a Smith machine or a loaded barbell for this version. Either wrap the bar with a pad or place a thickly folded towel over your thighs for comfort while performing this movement. Place a calf block, step, or weight plates below for the balls of your feet and fix your knees under the free weight or Smith bar. For the Smith machine version, lift the weight and then unhook from the rack (it is also a good idea to set the safety pins just in case). For the free weight version have your partner place the loaded barbell across your thighs and keep your hands on the bar for stability and safety. Perform the movement as stated above.

Leg press calf raises: Another great overall mass builder is the leg press calf raise. Normally performed on a 45 degree angle leg sled, (or machine leg press) these calf raises are convenient to do at most gyms when the traditional machines are not available. The trick to make these a bit different than the other versions we have discussed is to keep close to a 90 degree angle in your hips. This will stretch out the calves for an unbelievable contraction when done correctly.

Seat yourself in a leg press and place your feet about shoulder width apart with a slight bend in the knees – as discussed with standing calf raises. Lower the weight for a complete stretch and then reverse the weight under control for an intense contraction.

Important note: Many will load up the weight and do partial movements (the biggest mistake in calf training). Make sure the load is challenging, but not too heavy where you find yourself only lifting the weight half way up. Full extension and full contraction only.

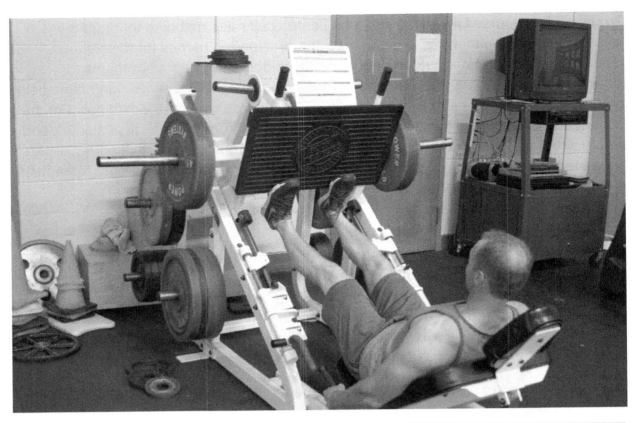

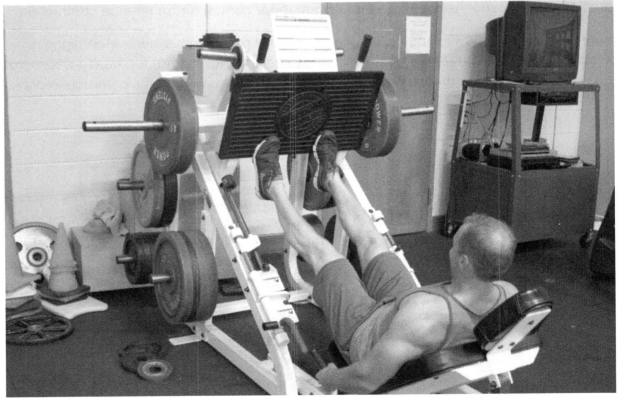

Tip: Another old-school movement that mimics the leg press version is the donkey calf raise. You may have seen pictures and video footage of Arnold and Franco doing these back in the Golden Era of bodybuilding. All you need for these is a calf block and a brave friend or two. Simply stand on the calf block with the balls of your feet (as in standing calf raises), bend over at the hips about 90 degrees and rest your arms on a bench or Smith machine bar. Your partner will climb onto your back to add resistance while performing the movement - straight legs, full extension, and full contraction.

Single leg calf raises: One of the best calf builders is a little-used gem called the single leg calf raise. It is very hard to find anyone performing these, but if you choose to, you will add strength and balance to your lower leg arsenal. Why? Because many times individuals are not reaching their full potential due to a strength and development imbalance in the lower legs. Once this is corrected, you can move ahead and start adding mass to your calves without compensating for one side or the other.

These can be performed with or without a dumbbell in hand (if you are new to this exercise it is recommended to start without a dumbbell to master the movement). Find a calf block and set one foot up as in the standing calf raise (straight leg, slight bend in the knee, back straight). If you are using a dumbbell, hold the weight on the side of the working leg, hold an upright for stability and perform the movement with strict from (stretch completely and rise all the way up on the ball of your foot for a full contraction). Switch feet and repeat.

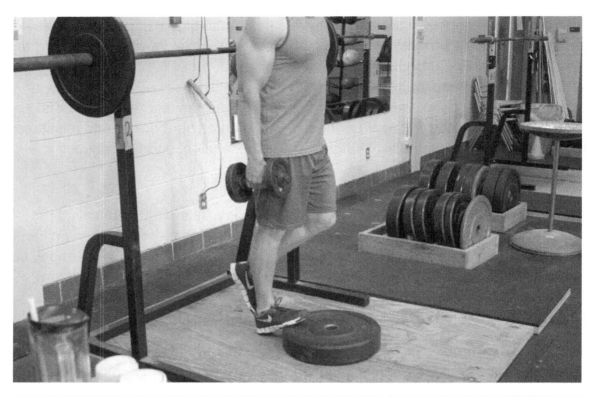

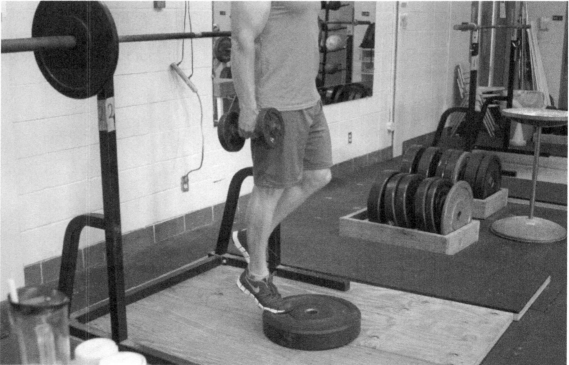

Tip: If you find yourself performing more reps with one leg than the other (which is extremely common), do a few forced reps with the weak leg. With your non-weight bearing hand, help yourself with a few more reps for the weak leg by pulling up a bit on the upright you are holding onto. The burn will be intense, but you will soon bring balance to that area.

Tibialis raises: A much forgotten (or ignored) exercise in the gym is the tibialis raise. Mainly reserved for runners, this movement will not only add mass to the front of the lower leg but will also help strengthen that area by developing balance to the antagonistic (opposite) area to the calf muscles. This, in turn, will enhance the performance and reduce injury to all of the lower leg muscles resulting in a more balanced physique.

Simply place your heels on a calf block and drop your feet for a stretch. Rise up (dorsi flex) on your heels while trying to point your toes to the ceiling above. No weight will be needed for this movement as you may find that this area may be a newly discovered weak point. Try not to rock back and forth – keep the form strict and feel the burn!

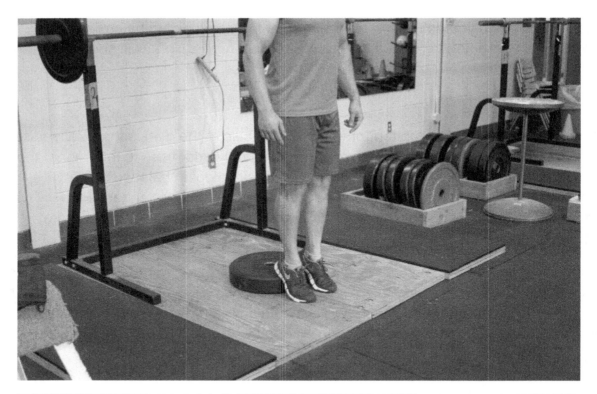

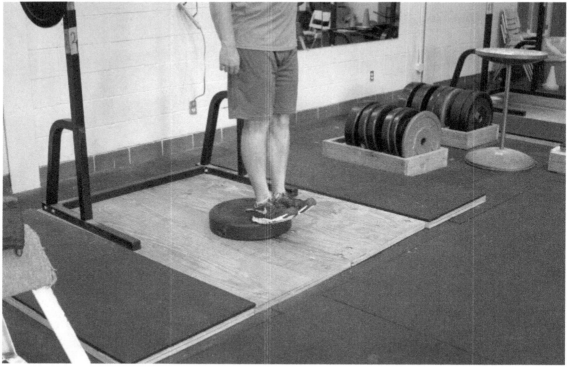

The Abdominals

One of the most sought-after body parts ever are abdominals. It seems everybody wants them, but few have them. Many toil away in the gym with sit-up after sit-up and crunch after crunch only to face sore abs and a declining motivation. Others don't worry at all about their abs and neglect training them all together. They are many times seen as an afterthought, tacked onto the end of a session only to be undertrained with little or no focus.

The abdominal area, midsection or core comprises of some significant functioning muscles. Not only does the midsection provide core stability and balance, it also aids in other lifts by redirecting pressure and stabilizing the entire trunk. By having the abs strong, the body can put more focus and energy toward a squat, for example, and hold in the pressure generated much like a weight belt. Next time you are bench pressing flex your abs slightly and keep them tight throughout the lift – you will be surprised at the help you receive from your abs during both portions of the movement.

So not only are the abs a significant factor in actual function in relation to other movements in your routines, but they can also be an unofficial barometer when it comes to being lean and proportionate. Aesthetically speaking, the mind draws instantly to the abdominal region as they should present a balanced and proportionate physique. A ripped midsection also signifies that the athlete is in superior conditioning and helps to display the coveted V-taper.

Along with a sound eating plan and a comprehensive training regimen sculpted, ripped-up abs can become a reality. Although this chapter will focus on the actual training regimen, creating an impressive midsection takes a very extensive eating component as well. One cannot do countless sit-ups and leg lifts every day and expect dramatic results. No other body part requires such discipline to develop, but once they are uncovered and for all to see they are a sight to behold.

Anatomy and function

The muscles of the abdominals comprise of several areas that flex, extend, twist and stabilize the trunk area. They sit on the front sides of the lower torso originating along the ribcage and attaching along the pelvis. Let's look at each muscle and its function.

Rectus abdominus: This is the coveted "six-pack" muscle – although it has more than six heads. This muscle flexes the spine and brings the ribcage and pelvis closer together.

Transverse abdominus: This muscle is a deep muscle of the core which lies beneath the other muscles that is essential for trunk stability.

Internal and external obliques: These are diagonal muscles that work to rotate the torso and stabilize the abdomen.

Ab builders

Now that you know a little about anatomy and function, let's delve into what makes outstanding abdominals. The movements presented are designed to get the most out of each trip to the gym. Remember to always use good form and not to use too much weight to compromise your safety. Remember when performing any abdominal movement be sure to execute each motion (concentric and eccentric) with steadfast control to avoid ballistic-style reps.

Upper Abs

Crunches and Sit-ups: The basic crunch is performed while lying on the floor with your feet flat on the ground, arms either crossed in front of you or hands behind your head and crunching your upper body toward your knees. Your lower back should not come off of the ground, just your upper torso. Crunch your abs and exhale as you come up. Squeeze for a second and then return without taking tension off of the midsection.

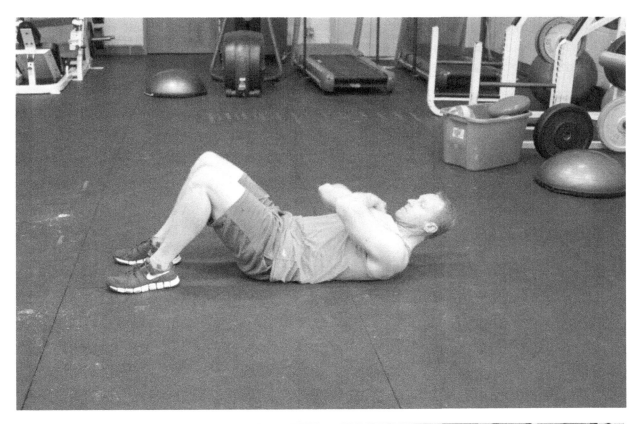

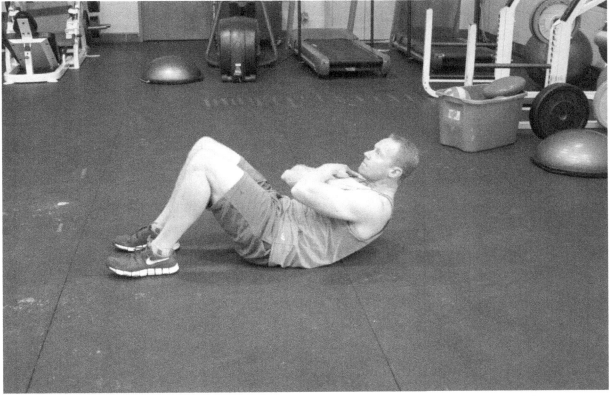

For sit-ups assume the same starting position then curl up your entire upper body into your knees. Uncurl and return to the starting position. Try not to use your lower back, instead let your abs curl you up.

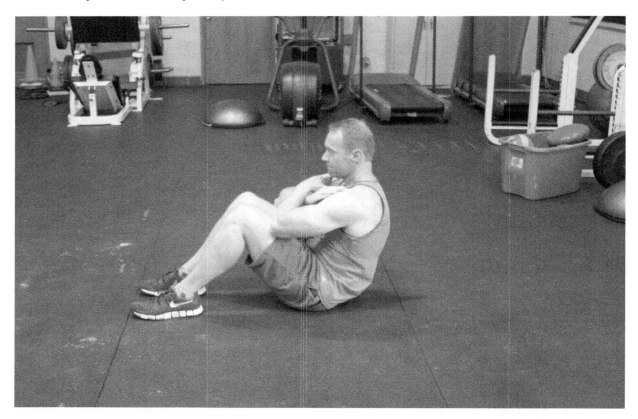

Tip: There are many forms of the crunch to choose from such as performing them on a flex-ball, feet supported on a bench, and weighted by holding a small weight plate on your chest. Another way to try weighted crunches is to stand against a pulley with your head toward a rope attachment and pull the weight up while you crunch. Make sure to hold the ends of the rope on either side of your head when crunching.

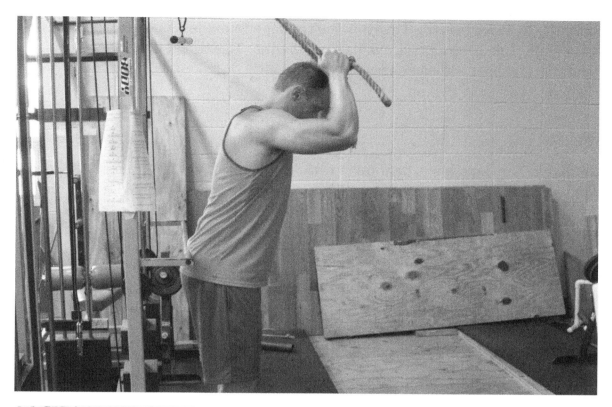

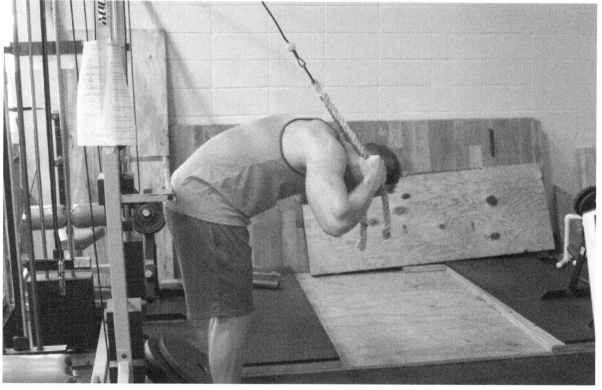

A great way to make the sit-up more difficult is to perform them on a decline bench and hold a weight plate on your chest with crossed arms. This would be a bit of a challenge, so try it with a weight you can easily handle first.

Lower Abs

Leg Raises: The leg raise is performed while lying face up on the ground with your hands slightly out to your sides palms down on the floor for support. With your feet together, lift your legs with a slight bend in the knees until they are just short of perpendicular to the floor. Lower to the starting position without letting your heels touch the floor and repeat.

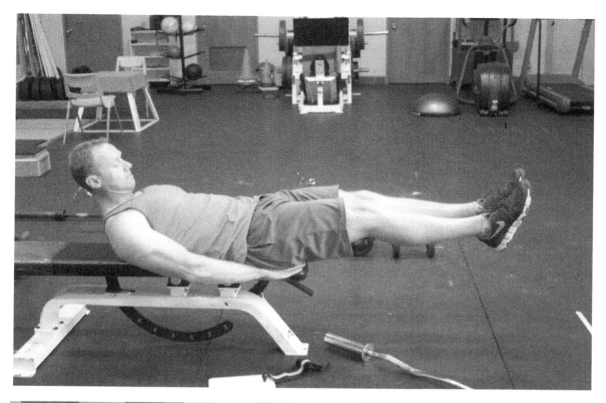

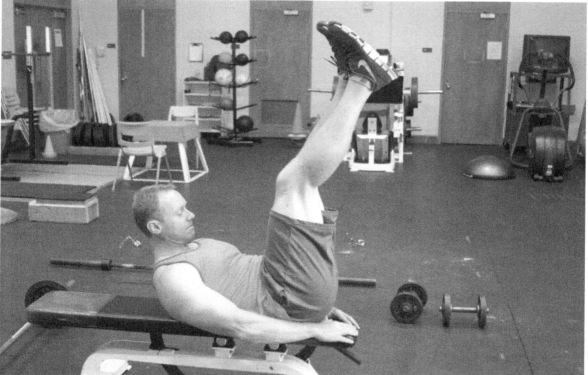

Tip: For a more of a challenge leg raises can be performed on a decline bench. This will require you to raise your legs over a wider range of motion for a more difficult and effective contraction. Hanging leg raises or knee raises are two more alternatives to really hammer the lower abs. While hanging from a chinning bar raise up your legs as in the lying raises and stop when your legs are at parallel with the floor and return. For knee raises bring your knees into you abdominal region until they are past parallel and squeeze. Lower and return as with leg raises.

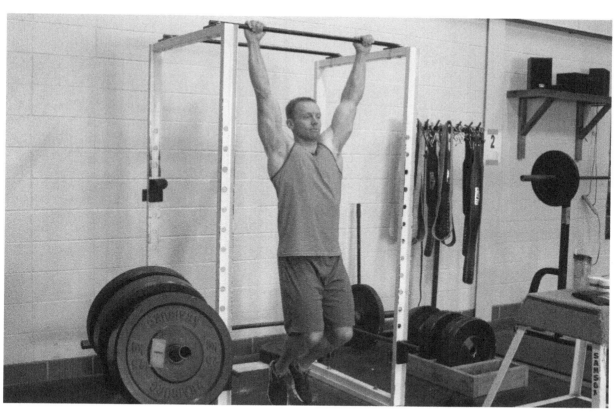

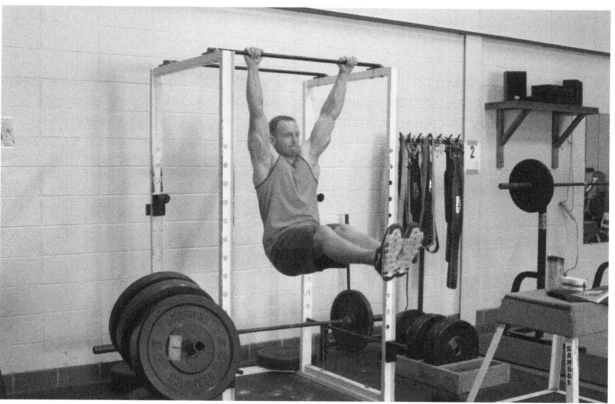

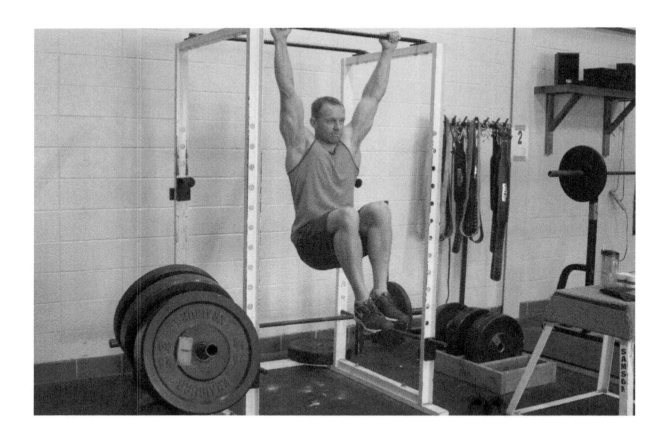

Obliques

Side Crunches: Lay down on the floor on your side with both hands behind your head - use a foot support if necessary to stabilize your lower body. Crunch up on your side while your hip remains in contact with the floor. Squeeze at the top for a second and then return to the starting position and avoid resting your upper body. Switch sides and repeat.

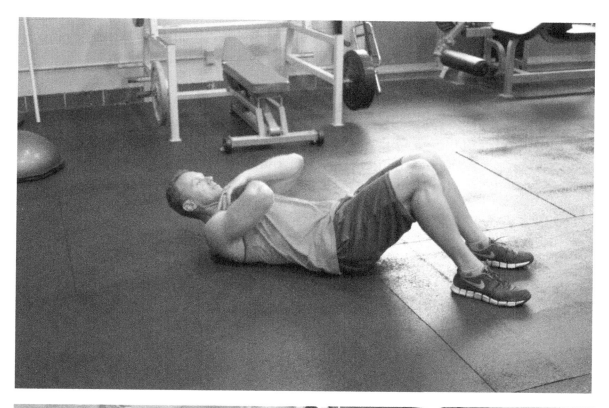

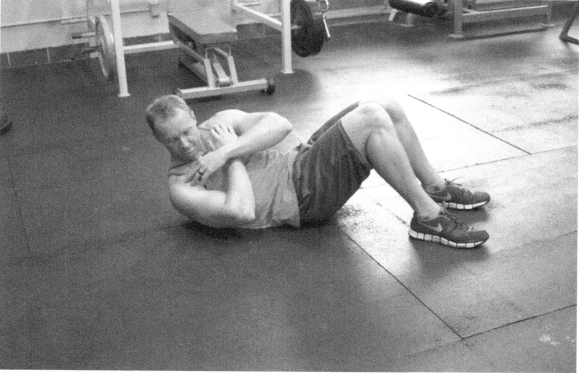

Tip: Side crunches can also be performed on a Roman and hyperextension bench. Simply position yourself with your feet and hip contacting the bench while your upper body is suspended. Perform the movement as above. This version will have those obliques screaming!

Bicycles: As one of the most effective ab exercises out there (especially for the obliques) the bicycle is not only challenging, but when done correctly, can grant you great overall ab development. Lie on the ground with your hands behind your head and your feet slightly off of the ground. Start alternating your elbows to knees. Twist your torso so that your left elbow reaches your right knee and then vice versa. Keep alternating while keeping your shoulders off of the floor. Squeeze the obliques with every contraction.

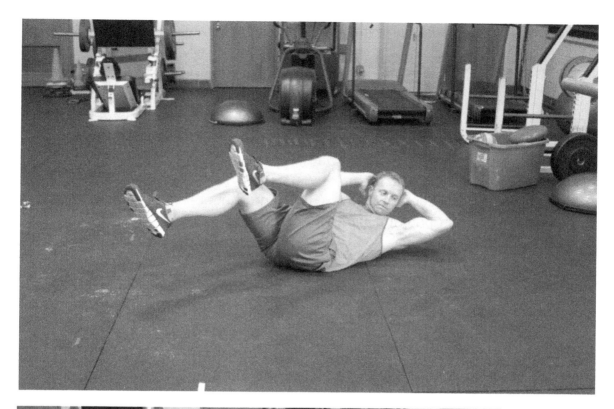

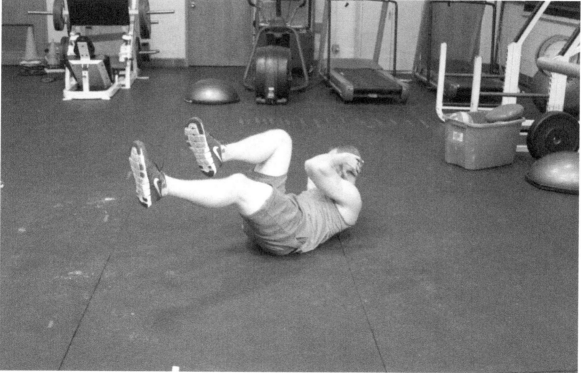

Tip: You can make this movement a bit more challenging and isolate one set of obliques at a time by focusing on one side and then switching over to the other. Just perform all reps for one side then switch and do the allotted number of reps for the other.

Russian Twists: This movement is not for the weak at heart. Seat yourself on a Roman chair or a decline sit-up bench where your upper body is suspended. Hold a weight plate or medicine ball out in front of you with your arms straight. You will begin to twist only your upper torso to one side as far as you can comfortably go then twist to the other. Keep twisting – but keep the movement somewhat at a slow pace. You do not want to jerk the weight around and injure your lumbar in any way.

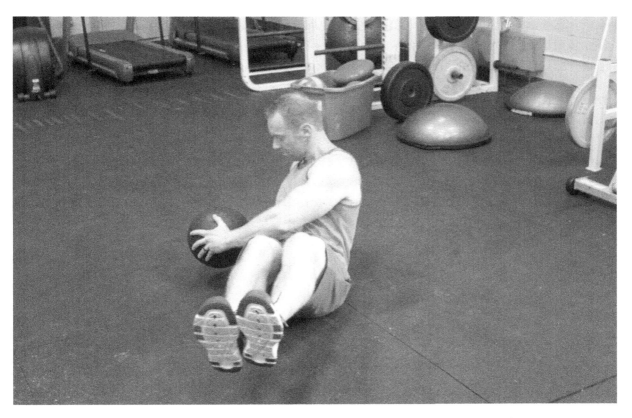

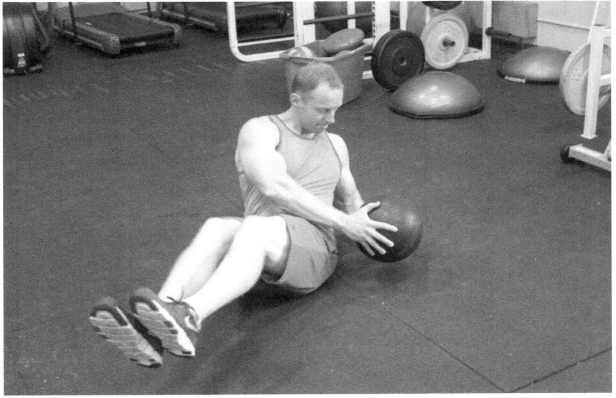

Tip: For those that find it difficult utilizing a weight plate or medicine ball with this movement simply clasp your hands in front of you and perform the exercise as usual. This will build up your strength so you may graduate up to using weight in the future.

Windshield Wipers: To really get to those obliques – especially the lower portion, try windshield wipers. Lie on the ground with your arms out to your sides - perpendicular to your torso. Bring your feet together and raise your legs straight up. Now, keeping your legs at 90 degrees to your upper body twist them to the side until they almost touch the floor. Raise them up and twist to the other side slowly. Again, jerking your legs will only make you more susceptible to injury be sure to use good form at a steady pace.

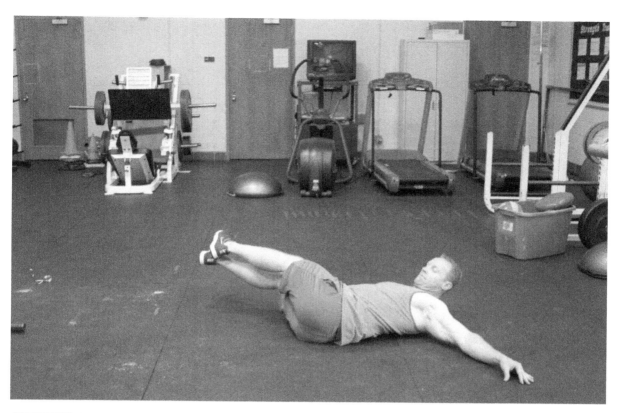

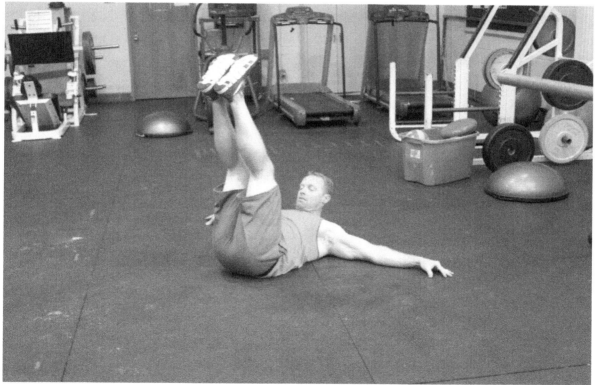

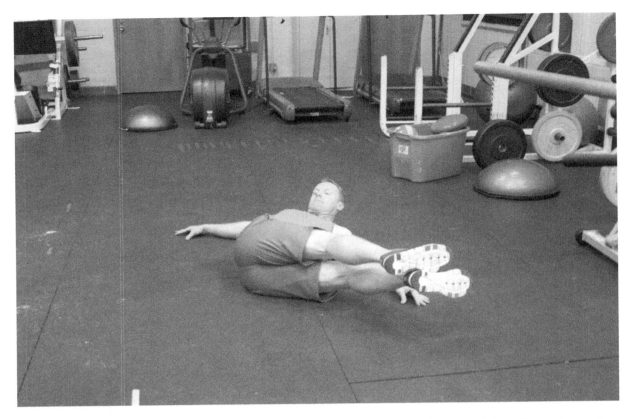

Tip: Once you have the basic windshield wiper movement down pat it is time to up the ante. Perform the movement as described above, but now place a small weighted medicine ball between your feet.

Overall core

Plank: Utilized as a standard for core strength and development, the plank is not a movement at all. It is a stability exercise used mainly to build the transverse abdominus. Simply assume a standard push-up position except hold yourself up by your elbows instead of your hands. Keep your stomach tight and drawn in slightly to activate your core muscles. Hold this position for 20 to 30 seconds and then rest – this will be counted as one set.

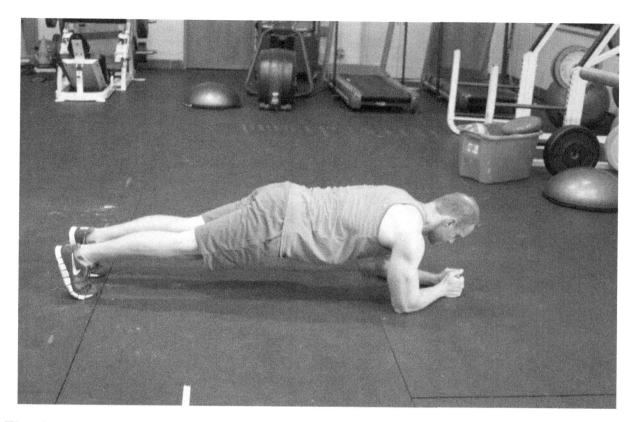

Tip: Once you reach a level of several sets of 30 seconds with the plank it is time for a new level. Have a partner place a weight plate (one that is at first light enough to handle) on your upper back to add resistance to the position. This new challenge will add even more strength and stability to your physique.

Side Plank: Much like the plank, the side plank works the core but on either side for lateral stability. With your body straight lie on your side while holding yourself up by you elbow and your feet together. You can place your other arm either straight down your other side or on your waste. Again, hold the position for 20 to 30 seconds and repeat for the other side.

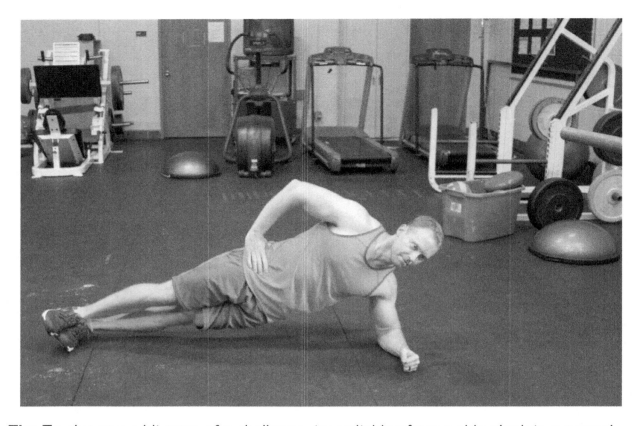

Tip: To give you a bit more of a challenge, try switching from a side plank to a normal plank over to another side plank slowly. Be sure to keep the body aligned and perform the movement in a steady, fluid motion.

Dragon Flag: As one of the more difficult movements to master, the dragon flag is the ultimate display in midsection strength! We've all watched Rocky do this one. While lying on a flat bench, grasp the sides of the bench by your head or the end above your head. Begin the motion by lifting your body up with only your upper back contacting the bench. While doing your best to keep your body in-line, lift until you are just short of perpendicular to the floor. This is a difficult movement to execute so go slow and try it with short lifts in the beginning if you do not possess the strength at first.

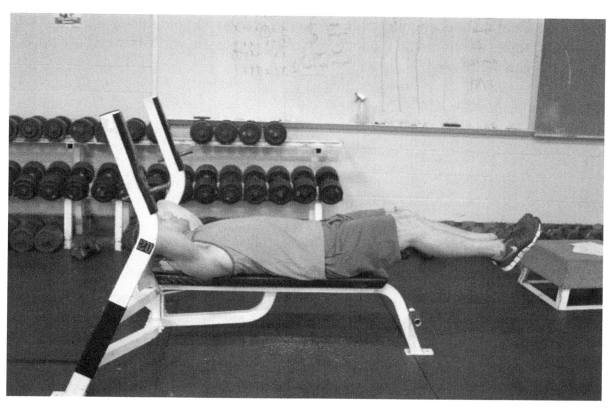

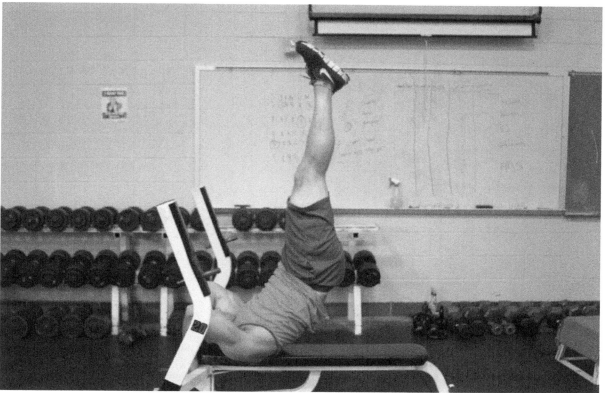

Tip: For the ultimate challenge try performing the dragon flag on a decline bench. This will take incredible strength and balance, but once mastered, you know you will have one outstanding set of abs!

Section 3: Goals and Training Programs

What about goals?

The main goal of the *Bodybuilding Basic Training Manual* is to pack on lean muscle. It is to reshape your body using weight training to put muscle on your chest, back, shoulders, arms and legs. It is to increase muscularity and develop a better built physique. If you've read this far then your goal most likely falls right in line with this.

As far as reaching this goal, it is imperative that you thoroughly understand that achieving the physique of your dreams takes hard work, discipline and time. Nothing worth having is easy. Remind yourself that every week, day, set and rep is another step toward your goal. Execute your plan, stick to it and, most importantly, believe you will reach your goal.

How do I set up my own training program?

Even though this manual clearly paves the way that will get you that physique you seek it is also important to know the "hows" and "whys" of a successful training program. Once your goal is firmly planted in your mind and you are ready to walk down the proverbial road, you need to understand such factors as frequency, volume, training time, duration, rest and program cycling and how they all fit together.

How much frequency?

These days pretty much most individuals train each body part about once per week. The way I see it that is only 52 opportunities to stimulate muscle growth per year.

Bear with me here.

Programs in this manual will utilize a training frequency of two and three times per week. Yes, you heard that right; you will train chest, back, legs and everything else two and sometimes three times per week. That will allow you 104 and 156 opportunities for growth over a year, respectively.

Of course it goes without saying that other factors such as volume, time and program duration will have to be closely watched as well.

How much volume?

Volume is the amount of total work done in a single workout. Many define volume as total sets multiplied by total reps (sets x reps) per workout. Some even throw in weight used per rep to get more of an aggregate total [(reps x weight) x per set].

Complicating things and doing math problems isn't why you're here. You need it done for you; you need to stop wasting your precious time with programs that don't work and get busy with one that will.

Now the volumes in these programs aren't something set in stone. I'm not here to throw math problems down your throat – I am here to take the guesswork out of your life. However, volumes are kept more on the moderate side of the scale due to the fact that your frequency is higher than the normal gym-goer's.

Instead of doing countless sets of chest exercises, for example, with numerous sets, you will have a more moderate number of sets so you can come back quicker and hit that same body part again. As frequency increases, your volume will decrease. Remember, more frequency equals more muscle.

How much training time?

I know there have been studies done on training length and peak hormone levels but for your sake and sanity you will hover around one hour of total training time. Some may be a little less, some a bit more. Simply put, if you can't get what you need done in around an hour, you are doing something wrong.

Additionally, one hour seems to be the best time frame for most individuals who don't have all day to live in the gym.

You can set aside the time, get in and get out. However, this time will be used effectively and efficiently so you can reap the best results.

What about program duration?

Most of the training programs in this manual will be of four to six weeks in length. In my experience, that seems to be the sweet spot giving you enough time to see progress but not too long to risk burnout. However, as the old saying goes, "if it ain't broke, don't fix it." If you're progressing nicely, why back off?

For most of you a four to six week duration on a specific program is a good rule of thumb for longevity, progression and motivational endurance.

What about active/scheduled rest?

After your four to six week stint you will go through an active/scheduled rest period. Active rest refers to performing some sort of activity or backing off of the intensity in your current program for a week to help rest and recharge your body before you crank up the intensity once again for four to six weeks.

This is advantageous for several reasons: it keeps you active enough to stick with whatever eating plan you are on, it keeps you mentally engaged regarding your goal and it keeps your metabolism in check.

Examples can include stopping several reps before failure on your current program, participating in recreational sports activities or trying out a new, low-intensity training program such as a circuit.

What about cycling programs?

This manual includes many programs to choose from so feel free to cycle on and off all of them. Even though most are geared for beginners, they all are effective for building real muscle. Just be sure to have that active rest period after every four or six weeks. The program templates will spell it all out to you.

Training programs

3 days per week full-body beginner programs

Purpose: A full-body program designed for the absolute beginner.

Duration: 4 weeks – take 1 week off after each 4 week period.

Frequency: 3 days per week with a day of rest between training days such as Monday, Wednesday and Friday.

Intensity: Don't take each set to muscular failure – stop about 2 reps before failure.

Progression: Progress to each new program every six weeks.

Beginner Program A

Exercise	Warm-up sets	Work sets	Rest (in seconds)
Barbell back squat	1 x 12	2 x 12	60
Flat bench barbell press	1 x 12	2 x 12	60
Medium-grip overhand pull-up	1 x 12	2 x 12	60
Standing barbell shoulder press	1 x 12	2 x 12	60
Floor sit-up	-	2 x 20	30

Beginner Program B

Exercise	Warm-up sets	Work sets	Rest (in seconds)
Barbell back squat or leg press	1 x 12	2 x 12	60
Lying leg curl	1 x 12	2 x 12	60
Standing calf raise	1 x 12	2 x 12	60
Incline bench barbell press	1 x 12	2 x 12	60
Barbell bent-over row	1 x 12	2 x 12	60
Seated dumbbell shoulder press	1 x 12	2 x 12	60
Barbell biceps curl	1 x 12	2 x 12	60
Parallel bar triceps dip	1 x 12	2 x 12	60
Lying leg raise	-	2 x 20	30

Beginner Program C

Exercise	Warm-up sets	Work sets	Rest (in seconds)
Barbell back squat	1 x 12	3 x 8	60
Lying or seated leg curl	1 x 12	3 x 8	60
Seated calf raise	1 x 12	3 x 8	60
Flat bench dumbbell press	1 x 12	3 x 8	60
Wide-grip pull-up	1 x 12	3 x 8	60
Standing dumbbell side lateral raise	1 x 12	3 x 8	60
Dumbbell curl	1 x 12	3 x 8	60
Close-grip triceps bench press	1 x 12	3 x 8	60
Floor crunch	-	3 x 20	30

4 days per week 2-day split beginner programs

Purpose: A 2-day split designed for the experienced beginner.

Duration: 6 weeks – take 1 week off after each 6 week period.

Frequency: 4 days per week with three days of rest per week. For example: Monday – day 1, Tuesday – day 2, Thursday – day 3 and Friday – day 4 with Wednesday and the weekend off.

Intensity: Go to muscular failure but stop there.

Progression: Progress to each new program every six weeks.

Experienced Beginner Program A

Days 1 and 3

Exercise	Warm-up sets	Work sets	Rest (in seconds)
Flat bench barbell press	2 x 12	2 x 8-10	60
Incline bench barbell press	-	2 x 8-10	60
Medium-grip pull-up	1 x 5-10	2 x 8-10	60
Bent-over barbell row	1 x 12	2 x 8-10	60
Seated dumbbell press	-	2 x 8-10	60
Wide-grip barbell upright row	-	2 x 8-10	60
Floor crunch	-	3 x 20	30

Days 2 and 4

Exercise	Warm-up sets	Work sets	Rest (in seconds)
Barbell curl	1 x 12	2 x 8-10	60
Close-grip bench press	1 x 12	2 x 8-10	60
Seated calf raise	1 x 12	2 x 8-10	60
Barbell squat	2 x 12	2 x 8-10	60
Seated or lying leg curl	-	2 x 8-10	60
Lying leg raise	-	3 x 20	30

Experienced Beginner Program B

Days 1 and 3

Exercise	Warm-up sets	Work sets	Rest (in seconds)
Incline bench barbell press	2 x 12	3 x 8-10	60
Flat bench dumbbell press	-	3 x 8-10	60
Wide-grip pull-up	1 x 5-10	3 x 8-10	60
T-bar or close-grip cable row	1 x 12	3 x 8-10	60
Dumbbell side lateral raise	-	3 x 8-10	60
Standing barbell shoulder press	-	3 x 8-10	60
Incline sit-up	-	3 x 20	30

Days 2 and 4

Exercise	Warm-up sets	Work sets	Rest (in seconds)
Standing dumbbell curl	1 x 12	3 x 8-10	60
Parallel bar weight dip	1 x 12	3 x 8-10	60
Standing calf raise	1 x 12	3 x 8-10	60
Barbell front squat or leg press	2 x 12	3 x 8-10	60
Barbell Romanian deadlift	-	3 x 8-10	60
Hanging leg raise	-	3 x 20	30

Experienced Beginner Program C

Days 1 and 3

Exercise	Warm-up sets	Work sets	Rest (in seconds)
Incline bench dumbbell press	2 x 12	4 x 8-10	60
Flat bench barbell press	-	3 x 8-10	60
Inverted row	1 x 12	4 x 8-10	60
Two-arm dumbbell row or barbell deadlift	1 x 12	3 x 8-10	60
Dumbbell upright row	-	3 x 8-10	60
Seated Arnold press	-	3 x 8-10	60
3-way crunch	-	3 x 20	30

Days 2 and 4

Exercise	Warm-up sets	Work sets	Rest (in seconds)
Incline bench dumbbell curl	1 x 12	4 x 8-10	60
Lying triceps extension	1 x 12	4 x 8-10	60
Leg press calf raise	1 x 12	3 x 8-10	60
Barbell squat	2 x 12	4 x 8-10	60
Dumbbell Romanian deadlift	-	3 x 8-10	60
Hanging straight leg raise	-	3 x 20	30

6 days per week 3-day split intermediate program

Purpose: For those wanting more volume and more training days per week here is a 3-day split designed for the intermediate trainer.

Duration: 6 weeks – take 1 week off after each 6 week period.

Frequency: 6 days per week with one day of rest per week. For example: Monday – day 1, Tuesday – day 2, Wednesday – day 3, Thursday – day 4, Friday – day 5 and Saturday – day 6 with Sunday off.

Intensity: Go to muscular failure and use intensity techniques sparingly.

Intermediate Program

Days 1 and 4

Exercise	Warm-up sets	Work sets	Rest (in seconds)
Incline bench barbell press	2 x 12	3-4 x 8-12	60
Flat bench dumbbell press	-	3-4 x 8-12	60
Push-up (optional)	-	3 x 8-12	60
Dumbbell side lateral raise	-	3 x 8-12	60
Machine or Hammer Strength shoulder press	-	3 x 8-12	60
Cable pressdown	-	3 x 8-12	60
Parallel bar dip	-	3 x 8-12	60
Superset: 3-way crunch and lying leg raise	-	3 x 20	-

Days 2 and 5

Exercise	Warm-up sets	Work sets	Rest (in seconds)
Standing calf raise	1 x 12	3 x 8-12	30
Seated leg raise	-	3 x 8-12	30
Leg press	2 x 12	3-4 x 8-12	60
Barbell front squat	1 x 12	3 x 8-12	60
Lying or seated leg curl	-	3 x 8-12	60
Hanging bent-leg raise	-	3 x 20	30

Days 3 and 6

Exercise	Warm-up sets	Work sets	Rest (in seconds)
Partial barbell deadlift	2 x 12	3-4 x 8-12	60
Close-grip pulldown	-	3-4 x 8-12	60
Inverted row (optional)	-	3 x 8-12	60
Bent-over dumbbell lateral raise	2 x 12	3 x 8-12	60
Dumbbell curl	-	3 x 8-12	60
Barbell curl	-	3 x 8-12	60
Superset: 3-way sit-up and lying leg raise	-	3 x 20	30

Body part specialization routines

The following are specialized body part routines to spice things up a bit if you feel you have a weak point or two. Some of these may include a bit more volume than the programs listed earlier, which is why you should only choose one or two of these specialized routines at a time.

Any one of these can easily fit into any of the programs in this manual. But be careful not to base your entire program around these routines as they would quickly lead to over training with the frequency specified.

You will notice that each body part specialization section has plenty of options such as upper pec emphasis, back-friendly legs and power routines to build maximum strength. Feel free to try any one listed regarding your needs such as equipment availability, current injury status or desired outcome. Also, don't be afraid to simply try something new and different. The only thing to gain would be more muscle!

Specialized Chest

Note: Perform 2 sets of 10-15 on the first movement for a warm-up with light to moderate weight.

Overall Pec Builder

Incline bench barbell press 3 x 6-10

Flat bench dumbbell press 3 x 8-12

Decline bench dumbbell fly 3 x 8-12

Mid-level cable crossover 3 x 10-15

Upper Chest Emphasis

Incline bench dumbbell press 3 x 8-12

Incline Hammer Strength or machine press 3 x 8-12

Flat bench dumbbell press 3 x 8-12

Low-level cable crossover 3 x 10-15

Lower Chest Emphasis

Decline bench barbell press 3 x 6-10

Hammer Strength or machine bench press 3 x 8-12

High-level cable crossover 3 x 10-15

Parallel dip 3 x 10-15 or muscular failure

Big Wide Pecs – Width Emphasis

Flat bench barbell press 3 x 6-10

Incline bench barbell press 3 x 6-10

Flat bench dumbbell flys 3 x 8-12

Dumbbell or barbell pullover 3 x 10-15

Chest Pre-exhaustion

Flat bench dumbbell fly 3 x 10-15

Incline bench barbell press 3 x 6-10

High-level cable crossover 3 x 10-15

Flat bench barbell or machine press 3 x 8-12

Superset Blitz!

Superset: Incline bench dumbbell fly and incline bench barbell press 3 x 6-15

Superset: Flat bench cable fly or pec deck and flat bench dumbbell press 3 x 6-15

Tri-set: 2-3 sets of 3-way push-ups to muscular failure

<h1 style="text-align:center">Specialized Back</h1>

Note: Perform 2 sets of 10-15 on the first movement for a warm-up with light to moderate weight.

Upper Lat Width

Wide-grip chins (total of 30 to 40 reps)

Barbell rows (to the chest) 3 x 8-12

Parallel-grip pulldowns 3 x 8-12

Hammer machine rows 3 x 8-12

Thickness

T-bar rows 3 x 6-8

Deadlifts 5 x 4-8

Wide-grip pulldowns 3 x 8-12

Lat pulls 3 x 8-12

Lower lat thickness

Lat pulls 3 x 8-12

Hammer machine rows 3 x 8-12

T-bar rows 3 x 8-12

Pulley rows 3 x 8-12

Overall mass and width

Close-grip pull-ups (total of 30 to 40 reps)

Barbell rows 3 x 8-12

Wide-grip pulldowns 3 x 8-12

Partial deadlifts 3 x 6-10

Pre exhaust

Dumbbell pullover or lat pull 3 x 8-12

Wide-grip chins (total of 30 to 40 reps)

Dumbbell pullover or lat pulls 3 x 8-12

Barbell rows 3 x 8-12

Pulley rows 3 x 8-12

Specialized Shoulders

Note: Perform 2 sets of 10-15 on the first movement for a warm-up with light to moderate weight.

Overall Shoulder Development

Military barbell press 3 x 8-12

Dumbbell side lateral raises 3 x 8-12

Bent dumbbell lateral raises 3 x 10-15

Barbell or dumbbell front raises 2 x 10-15

Barbell shrugs 3 x 8-12

Shoulder Width (Lateral Head Priority)

Seated dumbbell side laterals 3 x 10-15

Wide-grip barbell upright rows 3 x 10-15

Smith machine press 3 x 8-12

Leaning one-arm dumbbell side laterals 2 x 10-15

Dumbbell shrugs 3 x 8-12

Posterior Head Priority

Bent dumbbell lateral raises 3 x 10-15

Standing dumbbell side laterals 3 x 10-15

Seated dumbbell press 3 x 8-12

Cable rear laterals 3 x 10-15

Behind-the-back Smith machine shrugs 3 x 10-15

Power Shoulders (Strength)

Standing military press 5 x 5-8

Barbell upright rows 5 x 5-8

Barbell shrugs 5 x 5-8

Specialized Triceps

Note: Perform 2 sets of 10-15 on the first movement for a warm-up with light to moderate weight.

Overall Triceps Mass

Lying French press 3 x 10-15

Two-arm or one-arm dumbbell overhead extension 3 x 10-15

Rope cable pressdown 3 x 10-15

Inner (Long Head) Focus

Straight bar pressdowns 3 x 10-15

Close-grip bench press 3 x 8-12

Lying French press (straight bar) 3 x 10-15

Outer (Lateral Head) Focus

Rope cable pressdowns 3 x 10-15

Parallel dips 3 x 8-12

V-bar pressdown 3 x 10-15

Multi-Joint Only (Elbow Friendly)

Decline close-grip bench press 3 x 8-12

Parallel dips 3 x 8-12

Bench dips 3 x 10-20 (if using weight, use stripping method)

Cable Only

V-bar pressdown 3 x 10-15

Overhead rope extension 3 x 10-15

Reverse cable pressdown 3 x 10-15

Strength and Power

Flat or decline close-grip bench press 5 x 4-8

Weighted parallel dips 5 x 4 x 4-8

Bench dips with weight (optional) 2 x 5-10

Specialized Biceps

Note: Perform 2 sets of 10-15 on the first movement for a warm-up with light to moderate weight.

Overall Biceps Mass

Barbell curls 3 x 8-12

Seated dumbbell curls 3 x 8-12

Preacher bench curls 3 x 8-12

Biceps Peak

Incline dumbbell curls 3 x 8-12

Concentration curls 3 x 8-12

Hammer curls 3 x 8-12

Biceps Separation and Muscularity

One-arm dumbbell preacher bench curls 3 x 10-15

Concentration curls 3 x 10-15

Barbell spider curls 3 x 10-15

Strength and Power

Standing dumbbell curls 5 x 3-6

Standing barbell curls 5 x 3-6

Specialized Forearms

Beginner Forearm Program

Wrist curls 3 x 10-15

Reverse wrist curls 3 x 10-15

Intermediate Forearm Program

Reverse curls 3 x 10-15

Behind-the-back wrist curls 3 x 10-15

Hammer curls (optional) 3 x 10-15

Advanced Forearm Superset Program

Superset: Wrist curls 3 x 10-15/Reverse wrist curls 3 x 10-15

Superset: Preacher bench reverse curls 3 x 10-15/Cross-body hammer curls 3 x 10-15

Wrist-Friendly Forearm Program

Dumbbell wrist curls 3 x 10-15

Reverse dumbbell wrist curls 3 x 10-15

Hammer curls 3 x 10-15

Specialized Quadriceps

Note: Perform 2 sets of 10-15 on the first movement for a warm-up with light to moderate weight.

Overall Thigh Development

Barbell squat 3 x 8-12

Leg press 3 x 8-15

Barbell lunge 3 x 10 (each leg)

Leg extension 3 x 8-15

Outer Thigh Sweep

Machine hack squat 3 x 8-15

Walking lunge 3 x 10 (each leg)

Front squat 3 x 8-12

Leg press 3 x 8-15

Inner Thigh Focus (Tear drop)

Wide-stance squat 3 x 8-15

Leg extension 3 x 10-15 (lean forward)

Wide-stance leg press 3 x 8-15

Smith machine lunge 3 x 10 (each leg)

Pre Exhaust

Leg extension 3 x 10-15

Leg press 3 x 10-15

Leg extension 3 x 10-15

Front squat 3 x 8-12

Back Friendly

Leg extension 3 x 10-15

Leg press 3 x 10-15

Machine (selectorized) leg press 3 x 10-15

Leg extension 3 x 10-15

<h1>Specialized Hamstrings</h1>

Note: Perform 2 sets of 10-15 on the first movement for a warm-up with light to moderate weight.

Overall Hamstring Development

Lying leg curl 3 x 8-12

RDL 3 x 8-12

Standing leg curl 3 x 10-15

Pre Exhaust

Standing leg curl 3 x 10-15

Seated leg curl 3 x 10-15

RDL 2 x 10-15

Leg press (feet high) 2 x 10-15

Compound Only

RDL 3 x 8-12

Leg press (feet high) 3 x 8-12

Lunge 3 x 10-15

Strength

Glute/ham raise 3 x max

RDL 3 x 6-10

Seated leg curl 3 x 8-12

Back Friendly

Standing leg curl 3 x 10-15

Seated leg curl 3 x 10-15

Leg press (feet high) 3 x 10-15

Dynamic Stretch

Glute/ham raise 3 x max

SLDL 3 x 10-15

Lunge 3 x 10-15

Specialized Calves

Notes:
1. Perform 1 or 2 warm-up sets of 15-20 reps on the first movement
2. Rest only 45 to 60 seconds in between sets (utilize a watch if needed)
3. Do a different calf workout twice per week

Overall Calf Development

Standing calf raise 3 x 10-15

Seated calf raise 3 x 10-15

Single leg calf raise 3 x 10-15

Tibialis raise 3 x 10-15

Gastrocnemius Focus

Standing calf raise 3-5 x 10-15

Leg press calf raise 3-5 x 10-15

Single leg calf raise 3 x 10-15

Tibialis raise 3 x 10-15

Soleus Focus

Seated calf raise 3-5 x 10-15

Leg press calf raise (bent leg) 3-5 x 10-15

Tibialis raise 3 x 10-15

Seated calf raise 3 x 10-15

High Rep Blitz!

Leg press calf raise 3 x 15-25

Seated calf raise 3 x 15-25

Single leg calf raise 3 x failure (use bodyweight only)

Tibialis raise 3 x failure

Balance Program

Single leg calf raise 3 x 10-15

Single leg - leg press calf raise 3 x 10-15

Smith machine standing calf raise 3 x 10-15

Tibialis raise 3 x 10-15

Non-Traditional Workout

Smith machine standing calf raise 3 x 10-15

Single leg calf raise 3 x 10-15

Donkey calf raise (optional) 3 x failure

Smith machine seated calf raise 3 x 10-15

Tibialis raise 3 x 10-15

Superset Onslaught!

Single leg calf raise 3 x 10-15 (no rest between legs)

Superset: Standing calf raise with Seated calf raise 3 x 10-15 each

Superset: Leg press calf raise with Tibialis raise 3 x 10-15 each

Specialized Abdominals

Beginner Abdominal Routine

Floor crunches 2 x 10-20

Flat bench leg raises 2 x 10-12

Side crunches 2 x 10-12

Planks 2 x 20 seconds each

Intermediate Abdominal Routine

Hanging leg raises 2 x 20

Crunches on the flex ball 2 x 20

Side crunches on a Roman chair 2 x 20

Plank with weight 2 x 20 seconds each

Advanced Abdominal Routine

Low pulley, decline crunches 3 x 20

Bicycles 3 x 20 each side

Decline bench leg raises 3 x 20

Windshield wipers 3 x 10 each side

Plank/side plank combination 3 x 30 second each position

Advanced Superset Abdominal Routine

Superset: Decline crunches 3 x 20/hanging leg raises 3 x 20

Superset: Russian twists 3 x 10 each side/dragon flag 3 x 5 lifts

Superset: Decline sit-ups 3 x 20/weighted planks 3 x 30 seconds

Superset: Windshield wipers 3 x 10 each side/floor crunches 3 x 20

About Brad

A little about me…

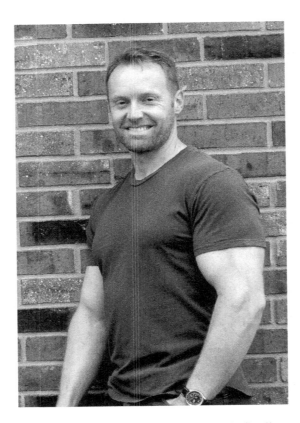

As not only a writer but also practitioner, I struggled with finding and executing the right methods of putting on muscle. Starting out as a skinny kid at 6'2" and 125 pounds, I sought out to find the answers to my challenges.

I earned my Bachelor's and Master's degrees in Kinesiology and am a Certified Strength and Conditioning Specialist (CSCS) with the National Strength and Conditioning Association (NSCA). I know, way too many acronyms!

I also competed as a drug-free, natural bodybuilder and have trained, motivated and consulted many clients from all aspects of life from the competitive bodybuilder and athlete to the elderly and rehabilitated. Having trained in commercial health clubs, wellness clinics, hospitals, university facilities and military installations such as tents, sand pits and old Russian bunkers I have also helped many with diets and eating habits as well as contest preparation.

I am also a veteran of the Air National Guard and proudly served in Saudi Arabia and Afghanistan. However, upon coming home from Afghanistan I was diagnosed with

Hodgkins Lymphoma (2004), an immune system cancer which my brother and father were survivors of prior.

I went through 9 months of chemotherapy before a full recovery and came back stronger!

I've written for numerous magazines and websites on the subjects of training, nutrition, supplements, motivation and everything cool. Currently I run my blog bradborland.com as well as write for other sites.

I have a precious son with my beautiful wife Courtney.

Thanks!

Brad

Made in United States
North Haven, CT
13 April 2022

18220882R00098